T0271494

Your Sexual Self

Also by Lucy-Anne Holmes

Your Sexual Self

28 DAYS TO EXPLORE, HEAL AND CELEBRATE YOUR SEXUALITY

LUCY-ANNE HOLMES

QUERCUS

First published in Great Britain in 2023 by

QUERCUS

Quercus Editions Ltd
Carmelite House
50 Victoria Embankment
London EC4Y 0DZ

An Hachette UK company

A CIP catalogue record for this book is available
from the British Library

HB ISBN 978 1 52942 404 1
TPB ISBN 978 1 52942 405 8
Ebook ISBN 978 1 52942 406 5

10 9 8 7 6 5 4 3 2 1

Designed and typeset by Clare Sivell
Printed and bound in Great Britain Clays Ltd, Elcograf S.p.A.

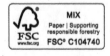

Papers used by Quercus are from well-managed forests and other responsible sources.

For You

CONTENTS

Before we set off, I just want to say that you are welcome here, wherever you sit or dance in the spectrums of sexual orientation and gender variance, whatever your experience of womanhood is or has been, and wherever you are in the world.

I hope this journey of sensual and sexual discovery is of value to you.

WHY WE NEED THIS BOOK . . .

There is something very exciting going on right now, and I want to bring it to you.

Women are reclaiming their sexuality, their spirituality, their pleasure and their bodies for themselves after millennia of male religious and state control. We're not in a multi-orgasmic utopia yet, and women in some parts of the world are able to accelerate this reclamation more than others, but something is definitely happening, and I believe it is essential.

It is our liberation.

For too long, female sexuality was presented to us by men. Men made porn for other men, so one learned about being a sexual woman via the male gaze and fantasy. This was exciting and titillating at times, yes, but it could also often be uncomfortable physically and emotionally, as though we were being asked to play a role that didn't fit us. And of course it didn't; we never chose it. 'You must be passive and desirable,' we were told. We were never asked, 'What do YOU desire?' 'Men have needs,' they told us. They did not ask, 'What do YOU need?'

I've been asking myself these questions for years, and allowing myself to play with the answers – answers that have often surprised me. For example, I have come to realise that I don't like penetration. Actually, let me reframe that: I love being penetrated, but I don't like being pounded. I don't want a penis – or anything else, for that matter – to move in and out of me . . . unless I explicitly allow it. This might sound simple, and I suppose it is, but realising this has been revolutionary for me, because for most of my life I believed that sex was about being pounded.

I also questioned my sexual orientation and discovered I wasn't entirely straight; I'd just been socialised to be so, and had therefore felt ashamed of, and ignored, my sexual feelings towards other women.

Best of all, I learned that I can give myself incredible sexual pleasure. I once had an orgasm that lasted three whole days, which I gave the understated nickname 'The Orgasm That Could Create World Peace' (because I think it could). This might sound a little 'out there', I know, but bear with me. When this orgasm was at its most intense and it felt as though I was spinning through space and time, in my mind I heard a voice that wasn't mine clearly say the words: 'This is the secret that was lost.'

Perhaps it's strange to be getting masturbatory messages from another dimension, but the words the voice said rang so true. Female pleasure *is* a secret that was lost. It took me until my mid-thirties before I even started to skim the surface of how amazing sex could be. Until then, I wasn't even sure exactly what my genitals included or what they were called. I definitely wasn't taught about female pleasure at school, and the porn I'd watched didn't end with women shuddering and moaning for ages while the guy looked on, jealous of the pleasure *she* was capable of. No. It ended with his jizz.

The more I thought about it, the more it seemed there had been a major cover-up. A sinister one. Clitorises cut from women, female sexuality and reproduction policed across the world. Women killed, mutilated, shamed. Repressed.

All that effort to suppress female sexuality made me start to suspect that female sexuality must be very powerful indeed. Surely, it's our duty to rebel and to investigate what all the fuss has been about? To explore this incredible force that so many cultures, faiths and men – and women, to be fair – have tried to frighten us away from.

I believe that exploring our sexuality, and owning it for ourselves, is radical. It's life- and world-changing. It is the most beautiful way to fuck the patriarchy.

Right, that's enough about me. *Your Sexual Self* is all about YOU.

It's for anyone who wants to claim and own their sexual self for themselves, who wants to ask questions about who they are and what they want, and who wants to play with and explore the pleasure they are capable of.

In it I bring you the wisdom of many great teachers, and the first-hand experiences of many people, including myself, but only you can explore your own body and find the answers that are true for you.

You are the star of this book.

You are unique, you are normal, you are magnificent.

I'm so glad you are here, rebel friend.

This is the secret that was lost.

HOW TO USE THIS BOOK

This book invites you to read, to write, and to do something each day. 'Read, write, do' sounds a little primary school for a sex book, so throughout the book I'll start with a quote and something to read for inspiration, and will refer to the other daily fundamentals as Curiosity and Sensation. You'll also notice the odd Creativity section, where you have the opportunity to get artistic with the process.

All the exercises in this book are offered with the same aim: that of you becoming acquainted with the glorious uniqueness of your sexuality, so you can explore, heal and celebrate this aspect of yourself.

It's important for you to know that there is no right or wrong way to complete this book. You may choose to use a journal for all your Curiosity and Creativity output, or you may prefer to keep a digital record. It definitely doesn't have to be done over 28 consecutive days, as the subtitle might suggest. You might like a particular day and want to linger there for a while whereas at other points in the journey you'll want to take a break. If so, please do. Go at your own pace. Listen to yourself. Trust yourself. Enjoy yourself. Repeat the Sensation section as often as you want. You may feel that you want to write poems or draw pictures in your journal. If so, how wonderful! Let yourself express whatever is looking to be expressed.

While this is a personal journey, you could also invite a trusted friend along. That way you can talk about it, remind each other about it, and also share some of your findings.

And please remember that while I am suggesting some things for you to do here, this is YOUR journey. It's always up to you whether you want to engage in an exercise from the book. If something doesn't feel right for you, feel free to skip the exercise. If you want to mix up the order because it makes more sense for you, then go for it.

If you find you have stopped working with the book for a sizeable length of time, I would urge you to question why this might be. You might be busy, which is understandable, but you may be resisting something in the process. Ask yourself why – and be interested in the answer. Then ask yourself, 'What do I need to do in order to carry on with this book and my sexual exploration journey?'

You might find this gives you valuable insights and allows you to continue.

My advice to you, now and always, is to be playful and curious.

The book is divided into 11 themes spread over 28 days. These are Your Love, Your Body, Your Sex, Your Intimacy, Your Pleasure, Your Desire, Your Power, Your Playfulness, Your Surrender, Your Sacredness and Your Vision.

Now, let's take a look at the fundamentals we'll be working with each day.

At the beginning of each section, I'll share some ideas for you to read and reflect on as inspiration. I hope these will inspire you to think about a certain aspect of your sexuality. I've tried not to go on too much! This section will always include a mantra, a quote and some of my thoughts, but you'll meet lots of interesting people here, too. I'll introduce you to some wonderful teachers working in the field of sexuality, and offer quotes and share experiences from people I've spoken to, and from those who have worked with me in workshops I have led when developing this course.

MANTRAS

If you've had a quick flick through the book already, you might have noticed that the title for each day is an 'I' statement of affirmation. I like to call these mantras.

The reason I have included them is that most of us have been 'programmed' with dodgy software when it comes to sex and the body. We discover that we've been internalising and repeating adages coined by angry monks in the Middle Ages, and slogans made up by ad executives in the 1990s, not to mention flippant comments made by family and friends when we were children. The mantras in this book simply offer opportunities for you to add some kinder, more empowering statements into your internal data mix.

When I lead the Your Sexual Self workshops, we start each day by closing our eyes and relaxing our bodies. Then we slowly say the mantra to ourselves, repeating it a few times and noticing our response to it. We are inviting these few words to bring us into a state of communion with ourselves.

Practise with me now . . .

'I am enough'

Place one hand over the other at the centre of your chest and take three deep, slow breaths. Allow big exhales to give you a sense of letting go – the same feeling you might get when you have completed all your daily tasks or finally got the kids to bed.

Close your eyes and slowly say, 'I am enough'. Allow a beat or a breath between each word. Repeat this a few times. Intersperse speaking with some big, slow exhalations.

How does it feel to say these words to yourself in this way? Weird? Calming? Exciting? Is it a pleasant experience, or is there resistance? What sensations can you feel in your body? Do any thoughts pop into your mind about it?

There's no right or wrong.

Simply notice.

The slower you take this (and most things!), the more you will feel.

CURIOSITY

On each of the 28 days there is a prompt for you to ponder and write about. This could mean thinking about a question, compiling a list, recollecting a part of your life story, or imagining something you desire. Write as much as you like in your answers. You'll know when you have written enough or when you still have more to say.

This is how we will process a lot of what we are experiencing and learning about sex, and where we will gestate all the lovely things to come. When it comes to sexuality and the body, journaling offers us a place to rest and access our inner wisdom.

I am a big journaler. I find that I don't really know what I am thinking or doing until I have pilfered a Bic from somewhere and put pen to paper. It is there on the page that I find myself or find my way through whatever I am facing. It is also where I find ideas and confidence. I can start journaling feeling down and worried, and end with an upbeat 'Go, go, go – you got this.' I still have reams of notes written when I started to explore my sexuality, as I pondered what I wanted, or mulled over my responses to various experiences.

Journaling has changed my life and the lives of numerous people. There is much evidence that journaling can help reduce depression and anxiety, and aid with recovery from trauma.[1] I very much hope that you find this aspect of the course helpful.

Practise with me now . . .

Why now?

Set a timer for two and a half minutes and write down your answer to this question: 'Why am I here, reading this book about sex?'

Now set the timer again and ask yourself: 'What do I hope to get from working with this book?' Let yourself write on after the timer has gone off, if you want to. You might find the questions quite similar, so don't worry if you answered the second in the first. Just carry on to the next section.

Notice how you feel about what you have written. Surprised? Intrigued? Fearful? Energised? Notice any thoughts that pop into your mind about your answers.

---

1 https://www.holstee.com/blogs/mindful-matter/5-science-based-ben-efits-of-journaling#:~:text=Studies%20have%20also%20shown%20that,-to%20reduce%20symptoms%20of%20anxiety.

How does your body feel after thinking about this?
Again, there is no right or wrong.
Simply notice.

SENSATION

Finally, each day includes an activity for you. This will be a meditation, a breath, touch or movement practice, or some other sensual exercise. In my opinion, this is where much of the magic of this book lies.

I share a lot about my relationship with my own body and sexuality in these pages, which you might find interesting or even inspiring, but my body is different to your body. The journaling exercises will give you profound insights into yourself and your behaviour, but bear in mind that until you begin to *do* things differently, nothing will change.

Sex is, by its very nature, more of a doing thing than a writing or reading thing. Sex involves sensation and touch, breath and movement, so we will embrace and experiment with these elements in this section. And sex creates a lot of feelings in the body, which is why, on this journey, we will be practising somatic experiencing, and asking ourselves more about how we are *feeling*, rather than what we are thinking.

The body *knows*. It knows our story and it knows what we need, and if we listen to it and allow it, it will lead us in the direction of its own healing and pleasure. Please: on this journey, and always, treat your body like a precious messenger.

Practise with me now . . .

Slow Down and Breathe

This is a lovely little practice which I do at the start of every Your Sexual Self session. Nothing happens before we've done this: no journaling, no exercises and no sharing of our stories and experiences. This is also how we will start each of the Sensation exercises in the book.

This exercise takes us from busy-manic-stressed mode to a more relaxed state. It's a process of consciously slowing down. It can feel like coming home.

Close your eyes.

Allow yourself an experience of slowing down and 'going within'.

Ask yourself, 'How comfy am I?' You might need to change position, yawn and stretch, get a drink of water, close a window, undo a belt or button. Allow yourself the space and time to tend to your own comfort.

Spend some time simply noticing your breathing. See how your body moves to take in breath and moves to release it.

If any thoughts come into your mind about other things, which they probably will, don't worry. Just take a moment to acknowledge them and then bring your attention back to your breathing.

Take at least three big breaths, with extended exhales. Allow the exhales to be audible, and make any sound that feels right for you. Feel as if you are letting it all go.

This long, audible exhale is a magic hack. When we consciously breathe in the way the body naturally would in a relaxed state, we send messages to our nervous systems to relax and be at ease. The vagus nerve tells the body that it's safe to shift from the sympathetic nervous system (fight, flight or freeze) into the parasympathetic nervous system (rest and digest).

Feel the gravitational pull down to the Earth. Notice how you aren't floating about in space, but are connected to Mother Earth. Notice all the areas of your body that are touching your seat. Now notice your belly, and how it moves as you breathe.

When you are ready, gently open your eyes and yawn and stretch if you need to.

HOW TO USE THIS BOOK

Notice how you feel now you have completed the practice.

There's no need to change anything.

Simply notice.

LET'S BEGIN . . .

YOUR LOVE

This part of the book prepares us for the journey ahead. It reminds us of our key principles of love, peace, safety and pleasure. This is where we practise moving our centre of awareness from the chatter of our busy minds to the sensations we feel in our bodies.

DAY 1

I am love

I just know that when I remember it, when it floods me,
as if from the marrow of my bones, as if from within the
blood stream, when the love that liberates, liberates me
it's the truest thing that has ever existed. It is the thing
itself. And time stands still, or never really was, or
maybe it's just that nothing can compete with this
truth, nothing can exist as intensely in any moment
as this love, including me.

Meggan Watterson, megganwatterson.com/

There's a lot of talk nowadays about how important it is to love yourself, and later we will be looking at how this is possible and what gets in the way of it. But for now, I'd like us to take a moment to remember simply that 'we are love'.

You, me, the fella who works in the corner shop, all of us. We are love; we just forget it sometimes. Our true nature is love. Our essence, our soul, our spirit . . . is love.

And why am I saying all this at the start of a book about sex? Well, because love is the engine that will be fuelling our sexual odyssey bus. I don't know about you, but I don't want my bus being run on self-flagellation or retribution or harshly imposed rules. That sounds shit. I want to have a tank full to the brim with the magic of love.

As we go through this book, we may need reminding to get back on the love bus, because every so often we could lose our way and hop on a fleet of other buses – the victimhood bus, the 'everything is pointless' bus, the bus of distraction (which take us down the wrong routes, stirring us up with thought patterns about how rubbish we are or how wronged we have been or how weird our breasts look).

It is then we will come back to the heart, and breathe. We'll remember that we aren't our thoughts, and that what lies beyond them is a peace, a gently moving stillness akin to love. 'I am love' we will whisper to ourselves. *I am love.*

Exploring our sexuality and sensuality is a way to experience in our bodies the love that is inside us. It gives us a glimpse of what we could achieve: our truly expanded self. It can allow us moments of magic and transcendence.

Great sex involves an openness of the heart. We must be welcoming of ourselves and our own experiences, and if another person(s) is also involved, we must open our heart to them too, and to what we could create together. But that's not all. I would say that in order for sex to enter the realm of the extraordinary, we must also be open to the idea that there is something greater and more mystical than ourselves at work.

I'm all about the love and the magic, and I realise that I'm hitting you hard with my hippy early on in our journey – but why not? We're all spinning around on a dying planet here; there's no time to be lofty and cynical.

How are you doing? Ready to board the love bus?

CURIOSITY

Two-Minute Love Blast

Set a timer for two minutes and start to list all the things you love: the people, the places, experiences, the activities, the smells, the tastes, the sights, the textures. There is no right or wrong here. No need to overthink it.

Notice your body now. How does it feel?

For another minute, write about how love feels to you and what sensations it creates in your body.

SENSATION

All-over soft-touch practice: the Bliss Touch

I came across this practice in the movie *Bliss*, when a sex therapist (played by Terence Stamp) recommended that a husband did it to his wife. That's why I call it the Bliss Touch. I love it being done to me by someone else, but I have found that I also love to do it to myself – as a precursor to masturbation and as a standalone practice to soothe me and add a little sensory something to my day.

I·start all my sessions with Slow Down and Breathe, followed by the Bliss Touch, *then* we say the mantra, *then* we talk, *then* everything else follows. A common response to the Bliss Touch is a moan of delight and a dreamy smile.

Touch is soothing. It activates the vagus nerve, signalling a sense of calm and safety. Touch also causes the brain to release oxytocin, the love hormone, that gives us that warm fuzzy feeling.

Place one hand over the other at the centre of your chest, close your eyes and go within. Feel yourself consciously slowing down. Take three deep, slow breaths with audible exhales. Let these big exhales give you the sense of letting it all go.

Now start to gently wiggle your fingers. Slowly move your hands to the top of your head, touching your head/hair as lightly as possible.

Continuing to use this feather-light touch, *very slowly* move your fingertips down and over your whole body. Trace a feather-light touch slowly down over your forehead, eyes, cheeks, ears, lips, then your neck, shoulders, breasts and so on down to your feet.

You might find that you are holding your breath: try to include big, slow, deep exhales as you carry out this practice.

If you come to a place on your body that feels particularly good, or interesting, allow your fingers to rest there for a breath or two. If thoughts pop into your head about other things, don't worry. Simply take a moment to acknowledge the thought then bring your attention back to the feeling of the feather touch.

When you have reached your feet, bring your hands slowly back up to rest, one over the other, in the centre of your chest again.

Notice your breathing. Notice how you feel, having done the practice.

Remember, there is no right or wrong.

Simply notice.

DAY 2

I am peace

The glorification of busy will destroy us. Without space for healing, without time for reflection, without an opportunity to surrender, we risk a complete disconnect from the authentic self . . . To notice our breath, our bodies, our feelings. To step back from the fires of overwhelm and remember ourselves. It may feel counter-intuitive in a culture that is speed-addicted, but the slower we move, the faster we return home.

Jeff Brown

Let's pause here and talk about speed. I must warn you, this journey isn't going to be a full-throttle sexual adventure. On the contrary, we'll be going veerry, veerry sloowwly. However slowly you're thinking we might go, it'll be a bit slower than that. It's a 28-day journey about female sexuality, and we don't even talk about genitals until Day 10!

As we all know, we live in a frenetic world, whizzing about on fast trains, with fast internet, doing fast banking, eating fast food, wearing fast fashion and worrying that we haven't got enough time. We're adept at wringing the joy out of most activities so we can get on to the next thing. If we're not too knackered, we might squeeze in a quickie or flick on some porn for a hasty wank.

Living at such a relentless pace can make us feel under immense pressure. When the Mental Health Foundation conducted a study of over 4,000 people in 2018,[2] it found that 81% of women had felt overwhelmed and unable to cope in the past year, and that 35% of women had experienced suicidal feelings due to stress.

Life in the patriarchal fast lane isn't so great for women. It doesn't work if you're on Day 1 of your period and you just want to be horizontal clutching your womb; it doesn't work if you've got morning sickness and a toddler in tow, or if you're menopausal and just want to tell everyone to fuck off and find a river to sit and cry by. Stress affects female bodies in such a way that it affects our sexual response cycle. It can inhibit the female reproduction system and cause a host of unpleasant menopausal symptoms by messing up the

2 https://www.mentalhealth.org.uk/news/stressed-nation-74-uk-over-whelmed-or-unable-cope-some-point-past-year

necessary work done by our adrenal glands. And when it comes to sex, if the sympathetic nervous system is activated, ready to deal with the threat it perceives must be coming with all this stress, then it's going to be unwilling to let the parasympathetic nervous system calm everything down so we can get our sensual jiggy on.

Fast sex doesn't really work for women, either. It can do sometimes, of course; I'm not saying it never works, because there is definitely a place in the shagging canon for 'the quickie'. The female body has the capacity for a whole range of incredible orgasms, but generally, the more time we take to relax and attend to the build-up of our arousal, the easier we find it to orgasm and the better our orgasms are.

In our breakneck world it's an act of rebellion to go at a leisurely pace. But good sex involves listening to the body, and listening to the body involves slowing down.

CURIOSITY

Explore this question in your journal.

When was the last time you felt comfort, peace and balance?
Describe how you felt, where you were, and what you

were doing. What was it, do you think, that made you feel this way? Can you remember how your body felt at the time?

You can write a few more examples as they come to you if you like.

Notice your body now. How does it feel?

SENSATION

#1 Do One Thing Super-Slow – much, much slower than you would normally

I love this invitation from my Brazilian somatic erotic educator buddy, Maria Eduarda Otoni. This is something she encourages all her clients to do when she begins working with them: 'Pick anything – making coffee, drinking coffee, walking on the street, and do it super-super-slow . . . I can't help but think "Isn't life beautiful?" when I slow it down.'

Slowing right down can make even the washing-up erotic. Warm water on my skin, sliding my hand across a smooth clean plate. Mmm . . .

Another wonderful practice to do very slowly is to cleanse your face or put lotion on your body. As my lovely friend Cat remarked when she did this, 'I spent all that money on bloody body cream – I can't believe I've never taken my time and enjoyed putting it on before!'

#2 Light Activation Meditation

This breathing visualisation meditation has become a bedrock of the sessions I run. I often do it before other exercises or as a gently transformative experience in itself. I love seeing people after this exercise, as they seem to glow.

You can spend ages doing it, as it is rather hypnotic, or you can do it quickly to make bus journeys a bit more fun. Please feel free to change it, add bits, play with it. Make this, and all the practices in the book, your own.

Slow down and breathe. Close your eyes and go within. Notice your breathing: how your body is moving to take in breath and release it.

Feel your gravitational pull down to the Earth. Notice how you aren't floating about in space, but are connected to Mother Earth. Feel all the areas of your body that are touching your seat. Notice your belly. How does the belly move as you breathe? Establish a relaxed breathing pattern in and out through the mouth, with long exhales. Allow yourself to feel as if you are letting it all go.

Now imagine that there is a ball of light at the centre of your chest, which I'll call your heart centre. This ball of light can be any colour or colours you wish – it can even be sprinkled with starlight. With every exhale, imagine that this light grows a little more dazzling and radiant.

Imagine that, as you exhale, it is as though you can send your exhale down inside your body, activating a column of light from your heart to your genitals. Your exhale activates this channel of light, and when you inhale you bring the breath back up the channel.

Spend some time sending your breath down and up this channel. Now we are going to activate a new column of light with our exhale. This time the exhale will travel from your heart up to the crown of your head.

Spend some time creating this new pathway of light, exhaling from the heart up to your head and inhaling down from your head to your heart.

Now we will join these two together.

Exhale from the heart down to the genitals. Inhale from your genitals up to your heart. Exhale from your heart up to the crown of your head. Inhale from the crown of your head down to your heart.

We will now activate one last area with the breath. Let your exhale spread out from your heart like angel or butterfly wings, encompassing your chest/breasts.

Then inhale back to your heart. Take some breaths to establish this new pathway. Now bring it all together.

Exhale slowly from your heart down to your genitals. Inhale from your genitals up to your heart. Exhale from your heart to the crown of your head. Inhale from the crown of your head to your heart. Exhale from your heart out to your chest. Inhale from your chest to your heart.

Repeat for as long as you wish. When you have stopped, sit in stillness for a while. Notice how your body feels now. When you are ready, yawn and stretch and gently open your eyes.

DAY 3

I am safety

I am able to regulate my system and become incredibly relaxed and breathe deeply and open up.

Angela, UK

On most journeys there is a safety briefing, and here I'd like to say a little word about triggers. A trigger is a stimulus that causes a painful memory to resurface. I feel it is important to say that this book may trigger some readers. The subject of sex, in general, comes with a big trigger warning. It can't not. The scale of violence against women worldwide is universal and devastating. We are the statistics. We are the survivors. And we are the daughters of survivors, going back and back for generations.

As you work with the exercises in this book, you might

find yourselves bumping into your wounded places, perhaps being jolted or nudged back to a place and time that wasn't kind to you, or to an incident, be it sexual, violent, medical or other, that you wish had never happened.

One legacy that traumas can give us is a sense of feeling unsafe in our bodies. Because of what has happened in our past, we may be living every day braced and ready for intrusion, yet we don't even know we are on high alert.

Our traumas can shrink what Dr Dan Siegel, a clinical professor of psychiatry, calls our 'window of tolerance'. The window of tolerance, put simply, is the zone where we feel safe and OK and are capable of having what can be described as normal brain/body reactions. It's the state where we are able to think and respond in an appropriate way to whatever we're navigating in life. Triggers and stressors occur, but we're still able to keep ourselves and our nervous system regulated.

But sometimes triggers and stressors can send us beyond our window of tolerance so that we enter a state of hyperarousal: fight-or-flight mode. This might result in us feeling anxious, agitated, panicked or aggressive. Or we might enter a hypo-aroused state: this is more of a freeze state where we zone out and become unresponsive. We can't choose which reaction we will have, because our brains take over in an attempt to protect us from these perceived dangers.

Today we are going to establish our self-regulation toolkit. This consists of some simple calming techniques which we'll explore in today's Sensation section. These were taught to me by Blaire Lindsay, a beautiful teacher, embodiment coach and trauma resolution practitioner based in the USA. We'll use these to help keep us in a relaxed state of arousal – a calm state. We'll also explore some exercises we can use in an emergency, when we quickly move outside our window of tolerance.

On this journey, let's remember how precious we are, and hold ourselves as such. Let's tread softly and take it slowly, and remind ourselves that we are here now, and we are safe in our bodies. We are safe.

CURIOSITY

Ponder the following questions in your journal.

How do I feel when I am in a calm state?
When I am feeling overwhelmed, what relaxes me and brings me back to a calm state?

Your answer should be a list of all the tactics you find useful.

SENSATION

The self-regulation toolkit

Below is a series of exercises that will help you find a state of nervous system regulation and relaxed arousal. They can be done any time as little meditative techniques to help you relax and centre yourself, or as go-to practices when you start to notice yourself veering outside your window of tolerance. I invite you to try them all. Notice how they make you feel, and which ones you particularly like.

1. Slow Down and Breathe

This one should be familiar! Sit down and give yourself time and space to settle. Feel your pace slowing right down. Ask yourself, 'What is going to feel welcoming to me in this moment?' And give yourself what you need. It might be coming to stillness, or it might involve some sort of movement like having a good shake or releasing a big exhale.

Close your eyes and begin to move inwards. Feel your gravitational pull downwards into your seat. Notice what parts of you touch the seat. Now, bring your attention down to your belly and notice what it feels like inside your belly. Take some deep breaths here with your awareness centred in your belly, exploring the movement and sensation of your breath.

2. Explore the question, 'What feels good right now in my body'?

Follow the steps above for consciously slowing down.

Locate a sensation in your body that feels good (if nothing feels good right now, then choose what feels OK or neutral). Simply be with this good or neutral feeling. Notice the sensation, stay with it, notice what happens when you stay with it.

We are so hard-wired to look for and focus on what is wrong that leaning into what feels good can feel like a radical act of rebellion. This is you resourcing yourself. This is you finding your anchor, your pillar of support.

3. Gently notice what is around you

Follow the steps in exercise 1 for consciously slowing right down.

Open your eyes and start to gently and slowly notice what is around you. Let your eyes widen slightly, as though they are alert, and track what is around you. Let your head, neck and hips slowly move and turn with your eyes as you look all around. Now, allow yourself to feel curious about one thing in your field of vision. It is drawing you towards it. Let your gaze rest there:

notice what happens in your body when you drop in and rest here.

4. Hold the body

Follow the steps in exercise 1 for consciously slowing right down.

Open your eyes, and slowly and firmly press a place on your body, saying, for example, 'This is my hand/shoulder/forehead' as you do. Feel the connection between your hand and the part of you that you are touching.

Do this to at least five places on your body.

5. Track your sensations

Follow the steps in exercise 1 for consciously slowing right down.

Shine a flashlight of awareness throughout your body and let it land on something that feels neutral or good. Begin to describe this feeling to yourself using sensation-based words, rather than emotion-based words. So, rather than saying, 'I feel sadness or happiness in my chest', explore the sensations you feel: 'I feel a dense heaviness in my chest' or 'I feel lightness and tingles'. Track three good or neutral sensations in this way.

DAY 3

Emergency calming techniques

Here are some recommended techniques for quickly coming back to a place of regulation.

Box breathing. I've lost count of how many people have told me that this is one of their go-to ways to manage moments of anxiety or overwhelm.

Simply breathe in for a count of four, rest for four, breathe out for four, rest for four, then repeat.

The five senses: 5, 4, 3, 2, 1. This is another popular go-to emergency calming technique.

Focus your sensory awareness in the present by looking for and noting:
- five things you see
- four things you feel
- three things you hear
- two things you smell
- one thing you taste.

Floppy noodle. Priestess and Temple Arts teacher Bliss Magdalena recommends the floppy noodle technique for people who find themselves quickly moving outside their window of tolerance. You literally wiggle around pretending your body is a floppy noodle.

Make it sexy. This method comes from Rosa, a Your Sexual Self alumnus. She has realised that her symptoms of anxiety – sweaty palms, increased heartbeat and breathing, pupils dilating, sometimes hyper-focus, sometimes confusion – are more or less the same as her symptoms of arousal, so instead of letting her body enter stress mode, she looks around for something sexy, or goes in her head and starts to fantasise. She finds it works almost instantly, and her anxiety is gone and forgotten and she is just horny!

CREATIVITY

Clare shared a prayer she had written; she says this to bring herself into a state of groundedness and calm.

Earth, support me and hold me up.
Air, caress me and give me life.
Fire, warm me and empower me.
Water, cleanse me and carry me home.

Write your own words, in the form of a prayer, poem, or whatever you choose, that you feel might help you

come to a place of calmness when you are feeling
overwhelmed.

DAY 4

I am pleasure

You see, in pleasure is freedom,
in pleasure is possibility.
In pleasure is choice.
In pleasure is creation.
And in pleasure is power.

Jonti Searll

The female body is designed for sexual pleasure. After all, we have the only part of a human body that serves no other purpose but to give us sexual pleasure: the clitoris. I want to let off some streamers here as I type this. It's quite a gift that nature gave us! Shall we make a pact here and now to spend more time strumming this little piccolo than, say, ironing or making pies?

Sexual pleasure is our birthright. I can't help feeling

that there should be more women lazing about on chaise longues, instructing their lovers to attend to their pleasure, or languorously tending to it themselves. As it is, women are far more likely to be seen getting a stain off the chaise longue than sitting on it.

As it happens, the statistics are grim when it comes to women's unpaid care work. Women and girls undertake more than 75% of unpaid care work in the world.[3] In 89% of households,[4] women and girls perform most household chores. My dear friend and tantra teacher Roxana Padmini had a realisation as a girl growing up in a Pakistani Muslim house in the UK that 'women are treated as servants'.

Most of us don't live lives where our own pleasure, sexual or otherwise, is a priority. It is more likely that we spend our time making sure that everybody else feels good and is looked after.

Our lives are busy and we're stressed. We also feel guilty about – well, everything. Studies repeatedly show women to be the gender that experiences intense feelings of guilt.[5] Surely life shouldn't be like this?

---

3 https://www.globalcitizen.org/en/content/womens-unpaid-care-work-everything-to-know/

4 https://plan-uk.org/blogs/unpaid-care-work-the-burden-on-girls

5 https://bradscholars.brad.ac.uk/bitstream/han-dle/10454/18058/40-34728.pdf;jsessionid=435B47C96990D22EFCB-9BE6B3F7CDBF7?sequence=2
https://journals.sagepub.com/doi/abs/10.1177/0022146510395023
https://www.redalyc.org/pdf/172/17213008014.pdf

The ramifications of this are ghastly for women's mental and physical health, and of course the effects bleed into our sex lives as well. 'Women don't prioritise their sexuality. They have to do everything else first,' sex therapist Anna Mrowczynska from Poland told me. 'They serve their children, husband, mother-in-law, parents – it's difficult for them to have sex before they wash the dishes.'

When we are so used to seeing women serving others at the expense of their own wants and needs, we unconsciously assume that the same rules apply to sex, and our sexuality becomes yet another area of our life where we put others before ourselves.

Much of our work throughout this book will be about moving pleasure up our priority list, remembering that we deserve it, that it's OK to seek it – and essential to experience it.

It is so important that we do this – not just for our own mental and physical health, but because if we don't stop putting everyone else's needs above our own then we will be modelling to another generation of girls that their pleasure isn't important, and that's tantamount to saying that their quality of life isn't important. That *they* aren't important. What would the world be like if women started to prioritise their own pleasure, and particularly sexual pleasure?

Let's find out . . .

CURIOSITY

Set a timer for two minutes. Write a list of the things that bring you pleasure. Now close your eyes and think of a time recently when you felt pleasure in your body. It might be a sexual experience that comes to mind, but it might not. It might be something that felt deliciously sensual – perhaps the warmth of the sun, a breeze, a soft fabric or water on your skin. Enjoy remembering this time, then write the experience down. Where were you? What was going on at the time? What sensations occurred in your body? Notice your body now. How does it feel?

SENSATION

I am going to introduce you to a wonderful teacher now, Betty Martin, and share an exercise that she places at the heart of all her teachings around pleasure, consent and touch. It is simply called Waking Up the Hands.

After the lips and the genitals, the hands have the largest number of nerve endings in the human body.

Hands love to feel things, and in this exercise we are going to let them. We tend to notice very little about our hands, but here we will allow them to feel good for no reason whatsoever.

#1 Waking Up the Hands

Sit down and lean back in your seat.

Pick up an everyday inanimate object. Register what this object is with your mind. Now use your hands to notice every detail you can about this object. Shape, texture. Are there hard bits? Soft bits? Rubbery ridges? Tassels? Smoothness?

Your mind will wander. That's what it does. Thoughts might come to your mind about this being a silly practice, or about what you might have for dinner tonight. If so, gently tap the thoughts away and bring your attention back to your hands.

Slow right down. The slower you move your hands, the more you will feel. Allow the experience to start to become pleasurable. Stay with those pleasurable feelings and settle into the relaxed state they bring.

Allow any feelings to arise naturally. Sometimes you may have an emotional response – joy, guilt or perhaps sadness. Just allow the feelings to arise gently; there's no need to change anything.

#2 The Pleasure Promise

You now have created some beautiful energy using your hands. Move your hands gently down your body and rest them lightly, one on top of the other, on your vulva. Allow yourself some long, audible exhales. Spend some moments here, simply connecting to this place of pleasure and power. Then say or whisper this little affirmation:

I claim my pleasure.

Take a breath between each word, speak each word on an exhale. Do this a few times. Afterwards, take some time to relax. Notice how you feel.

CREATIVITY

Write a story about a woman or a genderqueer/non-binary person who explores their sexuality. The story should be positive and have a happy ending.

For hundreds of years men have been writing stories about sexual women which have ended badly for them. Let's redress the balance.

YOUR BODY

Sex is a body thing. It's a mind and spirit thing too, yes. But above all – unlike crochet, say, or draughts – it is an activity for the whole body. In sex, the body is touched, felt, seen and celebrated. We can't bypass the body in sex, although we might try. This part of the book is about getting to know our bodies and asking them what they need. It is where we become a tender friend to, and guardian of, our bodies.

DAY 5

I am flesh

The body is not an apology.
Sonya Renee Taylor

When I was a child I loved doing cartwheels and handstands. I also really loved spinning, then closing my eyes and watching the coloured light patterns behind my eyelids. But by the time I was thirteen, I'd stopped spinning and instead sat crying in front of the mirror for hours. I had totally forgotten all the wonder and joy of how my body could *feel* in the sadness of how my body *looked* – something that only got more entrenched and entangled as I got older.

We bring the relationship we have with our body to the sex we have. We can't not. Unfortunately, through no fault of our own, it is incredibly common for women to have complicated – some might even say toxic – relationships with our own bodies.

It can feel frankly terrifying to allow ourselves, or someone else, to fully see our bodies, with their wounds and perceived flaws, so much so that during sex we may become tense, or we may numb ourselves with drink or drugs, or entertain an anxious inner dialogue about our inadequacies. Or we might have dissociated from parts of our bodies completely.

I get a bit ragey against the patriarchy at this point, because it feels to me that all of this is our inheritance from years and years of men having sanctioned domination over women and their bodies. Men decided what 'sex' was, and women were reduced to bodies that could be taken and owned – as well as judged for attractiveness, fertility and ability. Of course, times are changing and we're moving out of the worst of this, but we've still internalised it in such a way that we place an over-inflated value on how our bodies look and *should* work. This can mean that we can completely bypass our bodies' pleasures and needs.

Having a negative relationship with our bodies also means that women often accept crumbs when it comes to sex – when we should be getting the whole cake and being asked how we would like it served.

Sonya Renee Taylor was inspired to start a movement and write her brilliant book *The Body is Not an Apology* (a very good mantra!) when her friend Natasha confided to her that she was afraid she might be pregnant. When Sonya asked Natasha why she hadn't used a condom, Natasha said that her cerebral palsy made sex difficult enough, due to positioning; she didn't like to ask her partner to use birth control as well. It was then that Sonya found herself saying, 'Your body is not an apology.' This phrase has resonated with so many women who have heard it, as they too come to realise that they have been saying sorry for, and with, their bodies in a variety of ways.

Our relationship with our body affects the quality of sex we have and how equal and deserving of pleasure we feel. This is an important area to unpack, so in this chapter we will, very gently and lovingly, have a look at – and acknowledge – what's been going on.

CURIOSITY

We are going to shine a light on our relationship with our bodies. In your journal, write down the answers to the following question.

How did you experience your body at different ages?
Age 0–10
10–20

20–30

30–40

40–50

50–60

60–70

Over 70.

Notice any shifts from what felt like a positive experience of your body to a more negative experience, and vice versa. How would you describe the way you experience your body now? How would you like to describe the way you experience your body now? Remember that this is just your story *so far*.

SENSATION

We are going to stand up now and do a simple shaking practice. There is emerging evidence[6] and excitement about the benefits that shaking the body can have on our health, stress levels and in the processing of traumatic events. Our journaling exercise today may have

---

6 https://www.ncbi.nlm.nih.gov/pmc/articles/PMC4268601/

felt quite intense, so let's shake our bodies free from any tension that it may have left in the body.

The Shaking Practice*

Have a nice yawn and stretch

Stand with feet hip-width apart

Make sure feet are facing forward (not turned in or out)

Relax the whole body, keeping the spine straight

Begin to bounce very gently from the knees

Allow the knees to feel springy and light

Bring a gentle shake to the hands and wrists as well

Gradually let the bounce spread up the body, bringing the pelvis and hips into the gentle bounce/shake, then the waist, chest, shoulders, neck and head.

Close your eyes when/if that feels OK for you.

Allow the body to shake the areas where there is tension

Continue for at least 8-10 minutes, but longer if you are able.

Gradually let the bounce go and come to a stillness.

If you have time, finish with some light feather touch starting on your head and working down towards the centre of the chest.

Rest the hands there one on top of the other at the centre of the chest.

Notice how this feels in your body.
Notice any thoughts that may appear in your mind.
No right or wrong. Simply noticing.

*This is a standing shaking practice but for many of us standing won't be possible or comfortable, so find a position that works for you and start shaking from a place that works within your limits. Perhaps hands and wrists, shoulders, or wherever you are able to find a sensation of bouncing or shaking.

CREATIVITY

Create a piece of artwork that explores or represents your experience of having a body.

DAY 6

I am sovereignty

I have a body and it belongs to me.

Jane

Today is a day of reclamation: the day we reclaim as our own the voice that talks about our bodies. We choose sovereignty over our own bodies, recognising the power we have over what we say, think and do in relation to them, and no longer submitting to negative influences and powers that undermine this autonomy.

The mantra 'my body belongs to me' was coined by Jane in a Your Sexual Self workshop. I love its power and perfection.

Years and years of well-meaning friends telling her that she needed to lose weight had left Jane feeling as though her body was something separate to her, something that needed fixing. The words others had said about her body had become the words she told herself.

A funny thing happens when you start to examine your thoughts: you find that most of them aren't even yours at all. Let me give you an example. If I think of my hair, the first words I hear in my mind are 'dull, lifeless' followed by 'it's thin', 'greying', 'dry and damaged'. Now, these words definitely didn't originate from me; they've come directly from shampoo adverts on TV. A L'Oréal or Garnier employee has taken up residence in my mind without my even knowing. Hats off to them for such a successful ad campaign, but I don't really want them in my mind talking about my hair. I need to ask them to leave so I can create my own words for my hair. These would be something like 'my hair is fine'. Or 'There are 3.905 billion women in the world. We are all unique, we are all normal, we are all magnificent. All the hairs on all our heads are fine.'

But it's not always words that pop into your mind when you're thinking about your body; it may be images and comparisons too.

For about twenty years, I used to hate my breasts. Today, I find this a real shame, especially as they are so exquisitely sensitive – and they were much more handy than powdered milk and bottles for feeding my child. Breasts are pretty cool as far as parts of the body go – they're more interesting than elbows, say (and I have nothing against elbows).

Yet I hated my boobs from the age of eleven, when they appeared, because they didn't look like the pictures of boobs in the newspaper I saw every day. There used to be a daily picture of a topless teenager in the *Sun* newspaper while I was growing up, and I would overhear men make comments like 'Cor, look at the tits on that' ('that!').

I'm not saying it's a bad thing to see boobs, but when you just see one kind – big, perky, on teenagers – and they are in a family newspaper where all the pictures of the men are fully clothed, it sends confusing messages about what and who breasts are for. I carried deep shame about my boobs for years. I never really owned this part of myself because I thought my boobs were there for men to look at, and mine fell short. I thought *I* was the problem, not the pictures in the paper.

There are 3.905 billion women in the world. We are all unique, we are all normal, we are all magnificent. My boobs are fine. Pretty cool, actually.

Let's reclaim our minds when it comes to our bodies. Let's reclaim them from all the other voices that live there, from the people and companies that seek to tell us we're not good enough, that want to sell us stuff and subjugate us.

CURIOSITY

There are three elements to today's Curiosity exercise.

PART 1: Values

Set your timer for two minutes and answer the following question:

What principles do I have, or would I like to have, in regards to how I speak to others and about others?

For example, it might be very important to you that you speak kindly, carefully or with warmth and positivity.

PART 2: Investigation and reclamation

We are now going to investigate, and smoke out, anyone or anything that might be in our minds and speaking negatively about our bodies. We will do this by repeating a simple statement to ourselves and then listening for, and analysing, the thoughts that pop into our head in response.

DAY 6

Slowly write out the phrase 'I have a body' at least five times. Listen for any thoughts you have, and write them down. If no thoughts come but you feel there may be some, try writing 'I have a body and it's great' and/ or 'I have a body and it's beautiful'. Examine your immediate thoughts, and ask yourself where they might have come from. Another person? Media? Social media? The diet industry? Somewhere else? Could it be through feeling like you look different, having not seen yourself represented in media or daily life?

Decide whether you are happy repeating these thoughts and having these other voices in your mind. If you do not want these thoughts to be in your mind about your body, then in whatever way you wish – speaking? writing? kung fu? – tell these thoughts to leave your mind.

Now take some time to relax your body. From this calm place ask yourself what statement YOU would like to repeat about your body. Let this be your statement of reclamation. Repeat it to yourself like a mantra. And say it whenever you catch yourself saying words that are not your own.

PART 3: Going deeper

This can be a really difficult, important area, and you may feel that you'd like to do some deeper work here. If so, you might like to repeat the exercise from Part 2, but in a slightly more methodical, specific way. This can be done at any time – now, throughout or after the course. Below are some prompts for you to work with.

I have hair.

I have a face.

I have a neck.

I have a chest.

I have a stomach.

I have a back.

I have a bottom.

I have legs.

I have feet.

I have arms.

I have hands.

Take each statement and follow all the steps for Part 2 as before.

DAY 6

SENSATION

Today the first of our Sensation practices is to DANCE. Dr Peter Lovatt, AKA Doctor Dance, at the start of his lovely book, *The Dance Cure: The surprising secret to being smarter, stronger, happier*, says: 'We were born to dance. Dancing changes the way we feel and think and boosts our self-esteem.'

There's a huge amount of scientific research showing that dance is beneficial for mental and physical health. One study on conscious dance – the sort of dance we'll be doing today – found that individuals with depression or anxiety, a history of trauma, chronic pain, and a history of substance abuse or addiction reported the therapeutic effects of dance.[7]

If you still need convincing about how wonderful dancing is for our mental and physical health, then you might like to watch some of the many compelling TED talks about the power of dance. I recommend talks by Lucy Wallace,[8] who took dance classes into women's prisons in the US? She realised that most women in

---

7 https://www.sciencedirect.com/science/article/abs/pii/
S1744388121001390?via%3Dihub
8 https://www.ted.com/talks/lucy_wallace_dance_to_be_free

prison were suffering from some sort of trauma, and believed that physical movement would help them heal. And the talk by dance activist Jessika Baral,[9] who saw the positive effects of teaching dance to domestic abuse survivors. And the talk by classical Indian dancer Ananda Shankar Jayant,[10] who shared her story of dancing through breast cancer.

I'll stop now. You get the gist: dancing is healing and liberating. Let's do it!

#1 Dancing

In this exercise we move our bodies to music for at least a few songs, but ideally longer. If dancing around on your own feels a little alien to you, here are some guidelines to ease you into it. Start by playing some music you feel drawn to. You might like to try the exercise at different times of day and with different songs and types of music.

Stand with your eyes closed and listen to the music. Notice how the music feels in your body. Allow yourself to be drawn to a part or area of your body. Let this part

9 https://www.ted.com/talks/jessika_baral_you_are_how_you_move_healing_through_dance
10 https://www.ted.com/talks/ananda_shankar_jayant_fighting_cancer_with_dance

of your body move in any way that it wants to and that feels good.

After a while, become open to finding another body part to move with. And another, and so on.

For example, you may be drawn to some tension in your neck. Feel into that and let your neck move in whichever way feels good. Then you may be drawn to your hips, and want to circle them. After a while, you may notice that your wrists want to be shaken. And so on. Don't think about it too much; just follow where you are drawn to and what feels good. Remember your sovereignty. How does your statement of reclamation reverberate through your body as you dance?

#2 Apply Your Magic Body Lotion

Stop dancing and stand still. Feel the effects of your movement. Say your statement of reclamation a few times to yourself. Let the words sink into and settle in your body.

Now imagine that you have in your hand some magic body lotion that's full of your statement of reclamation from the Curiosity section. Massage this lotion into your whole body, thoroughly and luxuriously, then bring your hands to rest one on top of the other at the centre of your chest.

Spend some time now in stillness, noticing how you feel in your body.

DAY 7

I am gratitude

What we appreciate appreciates.

Unknown (but my friend Simon says it a lot!)

There is magic in gratitude.

Counting blessings as opposed to burdens (as Emmons and McCullough expressed it in their ground-breaking study into gratitude in 2003[11]) changes lives for the better. Mounting evidence shows that practising an attitude of gratitude makes us healthier and happier: it can also diminish acute pain, ease suicidal feelings, and even reduce blood pressure. According to scientists, gratitude is seriously good shit.

---

11 https://greatergood.berkeley.edu/pdfs/GratitudePDFs/6Emmons-BlessingsBurdens.pdf

And when it comes to the mechanism of our human body, there is a lot for us to be appreciative of. Without us having to consciously do anything at all, our heart beats. Our blood pumps. Our brain receives messages. A complex network of systems is at work within us all the time. We are truly incredible.

After acknowledging the biological miracle of the human body, we can also be grateful for what our body has endured, how it has healed, and all it has experienced. We should be grateful for all we can feel, such as cool sea water against our skin or a breeze on our skin, and all we can smell, such as bluebells in the woods. Be grateful for the way you resemble a treasured family member. We can be thankful for the way each part of our body tells our story, from our scars (from giving birth or from childhood falls) to the freckles your mother called 'angel kisses' and the hair your sister loved to brush.

Be thankful for the different parts of your body: the hands that caress, weave, cook; the nose that smells fresh coffee, mint, baking bread; the bottom, our personal cushion to sit on.

DAY 7

CURIOSITY

To start

In your journal answer the question:

What am I grateful for today?

Notice how your body feels. How do you experience gratitude in your body?

Main exercise

Write a thank you letter to your body.

List everything you are grateful to it for. Also – and this is important – be grateful for and excited about what you haven't yet received, for those things that your body is yet to do and experience.

You might like to do this on a nice card or paper.

SENSATION

I love the combination of the two exercises below. They form a lovely connecting, rejuvenating experience that can be used as part of a daily self-nurture practice or before other exercises or self-pleasure.

#1 Light Activation Meditation

This is the Light Activation Meditation you did in the Your Love section (see p. 31).

#2 Breast Massage

As I do for all the exercises in this book, I suggest a method below, but please don't feel that you have to stick to it. You may already have a breast massage practice that you want to follow, or you might like to try one of the many formats and techniques that you can find on the internet. Or you could simply follow your intuition, spending some time stroking and touching your breasts.

We'll all experience our chest areas differently. Our

breasts might be sore today, thanks to premenstrual breast tenderness or perimenopausal breast pain. They might be engorged from breastfeeding. We may have had surgery to enlarge or reduce our breasts. We might have lost one or both of our breasts.

Be mindful, and work gently around any soreness or scar tissue you may have. Whatever you do, the aim is to create a feeling of relaxation and warmth in the chest area.

We will be working with two types of simple strokes: long, straight strokes and circular motions. The key is not to rush, but to breathe and spend time on each stroke. This exercise can be done clothed or with bare breasts and oiled hands. Start by gently greeting your chest/breasts and connecting to this area with love. Cup your breasts tenderly and take some long, deep breaths.

Continue by touching each breast, using long, firm strokes that work towards the nipple. Work your way slowly around each breast, so that you travel across from the armpit, up from the belly, down from the chest and in from the centre of the chest.

Now use long horizontal strokes from right to left and left to right, starting underneath the breasts and working your way slowly up to the top of your chest then down again. Start with a small circular motion at the centre of the chest then gradually make the circle bigger so that the circular strokes gradually encompass your whole chest.

Now work first on one breast then the other. Start at the nipple and work outwards in a spiral motion. Do this for some time, then change direction.

Cup your breasts with your fingertips touching in the centre of your chest. Then stroke outwards over your breasts. If you sense that there is some other touch you feel your breasts or body might like, spend some time offering yourself that.

Spend some time in stillness at the end of the practice, noticing how your body feels now.

DAY 8

I am wisdom

I have a body. It is psychic, passionate, protective.

Rosa

It took me until my thirties, when I was on a very random road trip, before I began to look at my body as vehicle for experiencing sensation as opposed to an object that was supposed to look a certain way. This epiphany happened while I was travelling across Europe with two lovely German men. Now, these men were on a self-development journey and were part of a spiritual school that advocated self-inquiry – the practice of going within and exploring the sensations of the body. As a result, I spent many hours in a moving vehicle with two fellas periodically shouting, 'How do you feel in your body?' at me over the sound of German rock music. Something that turned out to be weirdly exhilarating.

Observing the sensations of my body was fascinating. So much was going on that I didn't have a clue about because I'd been hanging out in my manic mind all the time. I had twitches of arousal because I fancied one of the guys, a flushed feeling in my cheeks because I thought said guy really didn't like me at all, and there were contractions in my solar plexus because we were driving really fast.

Our bodies are always communicating with us. When we become curious about what they are expressing, they can give us a tender, fascinating insight into ourselves. So often, though, we skip that process. 'I have a headache' becomes 'I must take some paracetamol', rather than 'I have a headache. What is this telling me? Do I need to take a moment to slow down? Hydrate myself? Is there something my body needs? Have I had too much screen time? Is there something not right about my surroundings or life?'

As I mentioned before, it can be hard to prioritise and value listening to your body when our culture is so fast-paced and when we've been raised to focus our attention on how our bodies look and function rather than on how they feel.

A few years ago I had the pleasure of being taught by psychological activist David Bedrick. His book *You Can't Judge A Body by Its Cover* discusses some of the psychological work he undertakes with women around weight and shame. Very often the rhetoric around weight is 'Why can't this woman lose weight? She's lazy/selfish/not disciplined enough/not prioritising her health, etc.' But David marvels at the intelligence of the body, and explores what his clients are craving in their lives. He argues that 'understanding our hungers for love, power, freedom, respect, tenderness and more is critical to understanding our hunger for food'.

Our bodies are intelligent and wise. They seek to give us what we long for, and to keep us safe. They don't always get it right, though, and they need a bit of steering sometimes.

CURIOSITY

To start

Answer the following questions in your journal.

When do you listen to your body?
When don't you listen to your body?

Main exercise

Write a letter to you, from your body.
You might like to start as follows:

> Dear [your name]
> Hello, it's me, your body. I just wanted to say . . .

SENSATION

This exercise is in three parts, two of which you have done before.

1. 5–10 minutes: shaking (see p. 57) or dancing (see p. 66)
2. 5–10 minutes: lying down for Light Activation Meditation (see p. 31)

3. Intuitive Touch

Lie with your eyes closed. Allow yourself to be drawn to a part or area of your body. Bring touch to this area of the body in any way you wish and that feels good. If you find your body wants to move, let it.

After a while, when it feels right, release that body part and the touch there. Become open to finding another body part to touch. And so on.

You might first be drawn to tension in your shoulders and give yourself firm, kneading strokes there. When you let that go, you may notice that you want to gently stroke your neck, in a way that feels kind and sensual. Next you might feel as though you want to cup your vulva and rock your pelvis. If so, go for it.

DAY 9

I am reverence

I have a body and it nurtures my soul.

Carol

Today is our last day of the Your Body section, and we're going to mark it with a ritual to honour the body.

A ritual is a fixed set of actions and words that have a symbolic meaning. These actions and words, coupled with the intention behind them, can create experiences that transcend the ordinary and speak to our eternal soul self: little moments of depth and magic that connect us to love.

You probably already have several rituals in your lives. You might perform religious practices such as the Hindu morning washing and painting of the face after prayers. Other rituals might be more secular, yet still imbued with symbolic meaning: kissing your children goodnight, for example. At the start of his book *The Power of Ritual*, Casper Ter Kuile describes the ritual he has around watching the film *You Got Mail*. When he was a young gay teenager at boarding school, this film spoke to his deep need for meaningful connection, and soothed his feelings of loneliness. Now, as an adult, when those same feelings arise, he watches the same film – always with a tub of Häagen-Dazs pralines and cream.

When my mum was having radiotherapy for breast cancer in a faraway hospital, she and my dad developed a ritual of stopping at the same pub on their journey home. They would greet the waiting staff like old friends and order lunch and a glass of wine. It was their way of bringing joy to something bleak, of honouring life and pleasure.

CURIOSITY

To start

Answer the following question in your journal.

Can you think of any rituals you perform in your life?

Main exercise

Design a ritual to honour your body.

Decide how you would like to honour your body. You could do a ritual to honour your body's power, resilience and beauty, its capacity to feel pleasure and sensation, its ability to heal from disease or events. Or you could acknowledge your body after a transition such as the menopause, a birth, an illness. Or you could affirm your commitment to speak words of love to your body.

Decide what actions to include in your ritual. You might like to feature some of the following elements:

Music
- Adorning your body, perhaps with decorations or face/body paint
- Putting on a special or symbolic robe or garment
- Undressing
- Eating or drinking something special
- Looking in a mirror
- Lighting a candle
- Touch
- Movement
- Journaling
- Art
- Anything else you feel drawn to include!

Decide on the words you would like to say to your body in your ritual. There may be some mantras you have discovered here or written yourself that you would like to include, or passages written by someone else that feel meaningful to you. You might like to write something for the occasion – perhaps words of gratitude, an intention or pledge, a prayer, a poem or a song.

CHOREOGRAPH YOUR RITUAL

Decide where, when, how and in what order you would like to do the elements of your ritual.

SOME POINTS TO CONSIDER

Give yourself permission to be theatrical, playful, spiritual, meditative, creative, simple. Think about what you might like to do beforehand to make sure you're relaxed and focused on what you will be doing.

Fully welcome your spiritual self into this exercise and allow the practice to be sacred in whatever way(s) you wish. Connect to your gods, goddesses or ancestors who walk with you in love. There may be spirit guides, elements, angels or any beings of light in the unseen realms who are cheering you along on this journey.

SENSATION

Perform your ritual.

YOUR SEX

In this part of the book, we will be bringing your vulva and vagina lovingly into view.

We'll swot up on anatomy, reframe any damaging myths we might have learned about our genitals while growing up, and we'll begin to cultivate an attitude of reverence towards our sex organs – and ourselves.

BEFORE AND AFTER CARE

You'll notice that, from now on, as the Sensation practices begin to get more intimate, we will begin with a period of Before Care and end with After Care.

Before and After Care offer great opportunities for us to look after ourselves and to treat ourselves as important and precious. You might find that some of the techniques and practices we have done so far are useful for these times.

BEFORE CARE

Before Care is what happens before anything else happens. And it is crucial! Doing an exercise where you touch your vulva while making cheese on toast with the TV on in the background and your mum due to arrive in five minutes is going to be completely different to doing the same exercise in a softly lit room, with relaxing music playing, having just had a bath, meditated, and recited some words of intention.

Before Care is when we create the internal and external space for us to do the practices in this book.

In Before Care we can create a safe, loving environment for ourselves and our growth. This can be a simple, beautiful and empowering process in itself.

My own Before Care practice is detailed below.

My space. I make sure that windows are closed so there isn't a draught – and no one can hear me. I'll put on the electric blanket in the winter (I love an electric blanket!). I may tidy or move laundry piles or mess that will bug me. I'll dress in something comfortable/sensual/meaningful, get a glass of water, make sure my journal is nearby, then put on some music and light a candle/incense.

My body. I move my body, stretch out any stiffness, have a little shake and normally a dance.

My mind. I'll do the Slow Down and Breathe exercise, then the Bliss Touch all over my body.

My spirit. I'll generally be feeling pretty lovely by now. I rest one hand on top of the other in the centre of my chest, say a little prayer and make some intentions for the time I am about to have.

This can take anything from three minutes to an hour.

You might already have an idea of what you could do for your own Before Care practice. If not, let's take this opportunity to explore in our journals what this could look like.

CURIOSITY

In your journal, answer the following questions.

YOUR SPACE

How can I prepare my space so it feels safe and comfortable for me to do the exercises in this book?

YOUR BODY

How can I shake off the day and activate my connection to my body before I do the exercises in this book?

YOUR MIND

What might I do to calm my busy mind and relax myself before I do the exercises in this book?

YOUR SPIRIT

Which words of loving intention or prayer might I say or think to myself before I start the exercises in this book?

Use the notes you have made to write your own Before Care routine.

SENSATION

Do your Before Care routine.

AFTER CARE

After Care, by contrast, is what happens after you have done the exercises in this book. It is the time when we check in with, and listen to, ourselves. It is a time of tenderness and curiosity.

Again, our experience of doing a practice will be very different if we finish and immediately have to jump up to meet our ex-husband and jointly host a toddler's party in a soft play centre, for example, rather than spending some time in stillness, asking ourselves how we feel and noticing any thoughts that pop into our minds in response to what we have just experienced.

Journaling is a lovely way to connect to ourselves in an After Care practice, and this is a good way to ask ourselves what we need in that moment.

After an exercise, you might feel some or all of the following: hungry, thirsty, ecstatic, horny, emotional, sad, numb, jittery, smiley, angry. When you ask yourself what you need, the answer might be a nourishing snack, to practise some deep breathing, to go for a walk, to dance, sing, sob, have a shower, do some yoga, masturbate, drink wine, watch telly, eat chocolate . . . you get the idea.

It's important not to judge yourself for any of this but, rather, to be curious about what you are craving and why. Then you can mindfully give yourself a bit of what you need after a Sensation exercise, and allow this to become a self-loving ritual.

Your needs in terms of After Care will vary depending on how you feel, and you will get the chance to practise tuning into and listening to these needs as you go through the book.

During this After Care process – or at any point on this journey – if you discover an issue, whether it is sexual, emotional or physical, that you feel is affecting you and causing you pain or distress, you might decide to seek some help in a professional or structured setting. At the back of the book there is a list of organisations and types of therapy that may be relevant to you if this happens. (see p. 235).

DAY 10

I am sex

THE GREAT VULVA COVER-UP
In the early days
They were all over caves.
There was many a fanny on the wall!
The first ever work of art,
Not a dude or a heart,
But a lovely toe de camel.

A long, long time ago things were very different. Vulvas were everywhere. Archaeologists have found many images of vulvas carved in stone, bone and ivory throughout the Palaeolithic period.[12] These tended to be represented by

---

12 https://www.donsmaps.com/vulvastoneage.html

a circle or a downward triangle with a little line at the bottom. In fact, the symbol for 'woman' in the early written language cuneiform was a similar triangle symbol. The vulva was out and proud.

And the earliest-dated figurines that have been found haven't been of guys with big dicks. No, they have been of full-figured women with their vulvas on display. It would appear that women and their vulvas were seen as important and powerful.

But a great cover-up must have occurred, because when we get to the Greek and Roman eras, the men wildly wield their willies while the vulva disappears from sight, as though it's something to be ashamed of.

Nowadays, not only is the vulva generally hidden from common view, but the very words we use for the female genitals denote anything but pride and power. The German word for vulva, *scham*, literally means 'shame'. The meaning of 'pudendum' (a term for external genitalia) is 'thing to be ashamed of', and vagina means 'sheath for a sword (penis)'.

And yet here we are, alive at the dawn of a reclamation and remembrance of the vulva as a place of pleasure and power. There is more talk and awareness now about the female genitals than there has been for a long, long time. Once again, we are starting to see vulvas celebrated – even venerated.

But how do we feel about our genitals? Do we even feel connected to them?

CURIOSITY

To start

Answer the following questions in your journal.

Which words do you use for your genitals?
What words have you used in the past?
What words do you like and dislike?

Main exercise

Imagine you have met a beautiful new lover who you adore. They say to you, 'Tell me about your vulva and vagina. Introduce us, before I touch you there. I want to know everything so I can connect with this area in a way that will bring you pleasure.' Write down what you would say.

SENSATION

Yoni Breathing

Do your Before Care routine. You can be clothed, partially clothed or naked for this, whichever suits you. Find a comfortable seated position where your hips can be open – perhaps cross-legged or on a chair. Make sure you are comfortable.

Start to gently tilt your pelvis forward and back, making very slight movements, not exaggerated. Breathe in and out through your mouth. Don't worry about synching your breath to your movements. Your movements just help you anchor into your body and the awareness of your seat area.

When you are ready, gently move your awareness to your vaginal opening. Imagine your inhale and exhale coming from there. You may even start to feel this in your body. Now we are going to add another element to the practice. Bring the soles of your feet together on the floor: next we will open and close our legs with each breath.

On the inhale, open your knees and arch your back. On the exhale, round your back and close your knees. Move slowly, with slow breaths and long exhales. Invite in any other movement that naturally wants to occur. Keep feeling the breath in and out of your vaginal opening. Welcome a feeling of pleasure.

After about five minutes, stop opening and closing your legs, but continue to inhale and exhale through the vaginal opening. If your body wants to move too, let it.

At a time that feels right for you, let the practice ease and end. To finish, place your hands on your body in a way that feels good for you.

After Care

Spend some time in stillness.

Be curious. Notice how you feel in your body.

Notice if any thoughts pop into your mind. Don't try to change anything. There is no right or wrong. Simply notice them.

Now journal on (or think about) the following questions:

How was that experience for me?
How am I feeling in this moment?
What do I need right now?

If you are able to, in a slow and mindful way, offer yourself some of what you need.

DAY 11

I am power

I would get back from work, sit with a mirror and look at myself.
I thought, I want to see this beauty.

Wambui, Kenya

In 2021 in a Manchester teaching hospital 191 patients (twenty of whom were men) were given an anonymous questionnaire to answer. One of the questions they had to consider was: 'How many holes does a woman have in her private parts?'[13] There was also a diagram with seven annotated structures (labia majora, labia minora, clitoris, urethra, vagina, perineum, anus). Participants were asked to label as many structures as they could.

---

13 https://link.springer.com/article/10.1007/s00192-021-04727-9

Only 46% of respondents correctly answered that a woman has three holes: vagina, urethra and anus. And only 9% of participants correctly labelled the diagram.

The study was conducted by doctors in gynaecology and obstetrics who were concerned by the number of patients who didn't understand the nature of their medical problems: not understanding basic anatomy makes it very hard to understand conditions and, importantly, to consent to treatment. As therapist Kate Moyle says, 'There is empowerment in understanding.'[14]

So let's make sure this is one exam we'd all ace. Let's have a look at what we've got.

THE MONS PUBIS OR MOUND OF VENUS

I love sex educator Alix Fox's description[15] of the mons as 'a little pube-covered pillow'. It's the fleshy bit at the front where your pubic hair grows, below your belly and above your labia and clitoris. It covers the pubic bone at the front

---

14 https://www.theguardian.com/lifeandstyle/2021/oct/16/viva-la-vul-va-why-we-need-to-talk-about-women-genitalia

15 https://www.deccanchronicle.com/lifestyle/sex-and-relation-ship/181117/mound-of-venus-a-little-known-region-which-is-the-key-to-making-her-climax.html

of the body and makes a nice cushion if you are gyrating against someone. There are a lot of nerve endings here, so this area is lovely to caress, and comforting to cuddle.

THE LABIA MAJORA OR LARGER LIPS

These are the lips which, when your legs are closed, hide the clitoris and vaginal opening. They act as a shield for the inner sex organs. All labia are different: some are fleshy and bulgy, others are thinner and less noticeable, and everything in between. The outer side is where pubic hair grows. Here the skin can be darker, whereas inside the skin is smoother and paler. The labia majora can be very nice to stroke.

THE LABIA MINORA OR SMALLER LIPS

These are the hairless lips inside the labia majora. They surround the vaginal opening. This is a sensitive area with lots of nerve endings: labia minora swell with blood and darken when one is sexually aroused. Again, labia minora come in all shapes and sizes and are very sensitive.

THE URETHRA

The urethra is the tube that transports urine (wee) from the bladder and carries it out of the body. The urethral opening sits below the clitoris at the front of the vagina, in the vaginal wall. It's not easy to see or feel as it's really small. For some, though, this can be a very pleasant spot to stimulate.

THE CLITORIS

This has been referred to as the crown of the vagina. I rather like to think of the vagina having a crown. This is the only body part whose sole purpose is to give pleasure. Hurrah and thank you! What most people call the clitoris is actually known as the glans clitoris: this is just the tip of the clitoris, which is like a pea with a little hat on (the 'hat' is known as the clitoral hood – a crown on a crown!). It sits on the upper central part of the vulva below the mons and inside the inner labia. The rest of the clitoris is inside the body. It's a wishbone-like structure made of up of erectile (expandable) tissue which fills with blood. When a woman is aroused, it spans along and behind the labia and on either side of the vagina.

THE PERINEUM

This is also known as the perineal sponge. It is an area of cushiony tissue between the vagina and anus. This is a sensitive area, and you may enjoy being stroked here or having more pressure applied.

THE VAGINA

The vagina is a stretchy tube between the vulva and the cervix (the entrance to the womb). It is where menstrual blood and babies exit. It is also where a penis, finger, sex toy or tampon can enter. We call it a tube, but when the vagina is relaxed, its walls collapse in on each other, so that if you looked at a cross-section of a vagina, it would look less like an O and more like a W or an H in shape. When aroused, the vagina stretches and widens. This can be referred to as tenting and ballooning. Some places along the walls of the vagina can be very sensitive, especially after clitoral stimulation, so it is a very good place to explore. The vaginal walls are made of similar tissue and texture as the inside of the mouth.

THE ANUS

The anus, or bumhole, is behind the vagina. It opens to your rectum, and is where faeces (poo) leaves your body. It has loads of sensitive nerve endings, and some people get sexual pleasure from being stimulated here.

CURIOSITY

To start

Answer the following questions in your journal.

When were you last aware of your genitals feeling good?
What sensations did you feel?
What was going on?

Main exercise

Write a love letter to your genitals.

SENSATION

There are two parts to this exercise. They can be done one after the other or at different times, whichever you feel is best for you.

#1 Vulva Self-Study

Do your Before Care routine.

Now you will spend some time being curious about and exploring your vulva. You will need a mirror, small or large. You may like to have some oil so you can smoothly touch each part of your vulva. Position the mirror so that you can see between your legs. When you are ready, take off your underwear and open your legs.

You are simply going to look at your vulva and see if you can identify the places mentioned previously: the mons pubis, the labia majora, the labia minora, the urethra, the clitoris, the perineum, the vagina, the anus.

Do not judge or criticise what you see. Rather, foster an attitude of impartial curiosity. Gently close your legs when you feel the exercise is complete.

After Care

Spend some time in stillness.

Be curious. Notice how you feel in your body.

Notice if any thoughts pop into your mind. Don't try to change anything. There is no right or wrong. Simply notice them.

Now journal on (or think about) the following questions:

How was that experience for me?
How am I feeling in this moment?
What do I need right now?

If you are able to, in a slow and mindful way, offer yourself some of what you need.

#2 Vulva Gazing

In this exercise we are going to look at our genitals again. This time, rather than being objective, we will be taking an attitude of gentle reverence.

Do your Before Care routine. Then, when you are ready, gently reveal your vulva so that you can see yourself in the mirror. Taking long, relaxed breaths, simply gaze at your vulva.

Allow this to be a meditation. Imagine you are gazing at the most holy thing in the world. Spend at least ten minutes doing this. Then, very gently and slowly, close your legs.

Finish, as before, with After Care.

CREATIVITY

Make, label and decorate (if you wish) your own dia-gram, picture or model of the female genitals. This could be anything – a quick pencil drawing in your notebook, a glittery collage, a clay model, a bejewelled mosaic, a tapestry, a frilly cushion or aerosol graffiti on a wall.

I am magic

*Rejoicing at her wondrous vulva, the young woman
Inanna applauded herself.*

Inanna, Queen of Heaven,
ancient Mesopotamian goddess of love and sex

It is hard to imagine a part of the body that is more important, symbolic or magical than the female sex organs. It is
literally the doorway to life: a gateway from darkness into
light, a place of receiving and releasing, a place of transcendent sensation. It is power and pleasure on an almost
indescribable scale. You can understand why our ancestors carved it all over their caves.

But most of us have grown up in a patriarchal world,
without a single 'power of the pussy' fresco to be seen.

Instead, we have absorbed a gazillion messages that make us feel as if our genitals are something to be ashamed of, or even that they don't belong to us. The Bible talks of women's 'menstrual impurity', Femfresh[16] implies that we're smelly, 'your vagina is so big and baggy . . .' jokes abound, a US president says 'Grab 'em by the pussy', and plastic surgeons encourage us to buy a vulva like Barbie's.[17]

'Close your legs' was a refrain many of us heard during our childhoods, along with 'It's dirty', 'You'll go blind if you touch down there' and other clangers. Sophie from Iran, who I interviewed for my book, *Women on Top of the World: What women think about when they have sex*, spoke about rumours being passed from older girls to younger ones to scare them, such as if you touched yourself 'down there' it would leave a mark and you'd become unmarriable.

We were taught to leave it alone, cover it up, change it. It would have been nice to be told to rejoice, revel in and respect this area of our bodies. It's now up to us to reclaim our relationship with our genitals – and reframe it how *we* wish it to be.

---

16 https://onlinelibrary.wiley.com/doi/full/10.1111/1468-0424.12617
17 https://www.stylist.co.uk/life/these-barbie-pussy-labiaplasty-ads-have-been-banned-from-instagram/180950

CURIOSITY

To start

Answer the following questions in your journal.

What messages were you were told or did you absorb about your genitals as a child and as you grew up? What do you wish you had been told or taught about your genitals when you were growing up?

Main exercise

Write the following question in your journal and allow your genitals to answer you in the first person.

Hello, how are you doing? What do you need?

SENSATION

Read what you wrote in the above exercise. Now create, if you can, an experience where you give your vulva what it needs. Whether this means buying yourself some more comfy knickers or offering yourself genital touch in the bath, make it an intimate experience for yourself. Follow the steps of your Before Care practice to start. End with a period of After Care.

Extra Sensation Practice
(to be done any time you wish)

DATE NIGHT

This can be such a beautiful exercise. Regena Thomashauer, otherwise known as Mama Gena, at the start of her hugely successful book *Pussy: A reclamation*, explains how this simple exercise changed her life as it made her realise that women tend to have no idea of their own beauty, power and magnificence.

It can be done at any time during the course. It's nice to take your time planning this one and shopping for delicacies!

DAY 12

Prepare your environment as though you are expecting the most special guest in the world. How would you like your space to be for their arrival? What will you offer them to eat and drink? How will you prepare and dress for your special guest?

But YOU are your special guest!

Enjoy the beautiful space and treats you have prepared. Now stand naked in front of a mirror and notice all that you like about yourself. Then lie on your bed and give yourself sensual touch in whatever way you wish.

DAY 13

I am devotion

. . . and the women knead the dough and make cakes to offer to the Queen of Heaven.

Jeremiah 7:18

I find the above line in the Bible hugely exciting. What were the women doing? Who was the Queen of Heaven? What were these cakes?

From doing some research, I found that the Queen of Heaven here is the goddess Ishtar. Interestingly, she is said to be a later form of Inanna (who, as we learned in Day 12, loved her vulva). Ishtar was the Mesopotamian goddess of love, fertility, sexuality and war. She was elevated to the highest Mesopotamian pantheon of gods and was worshipped for almost 3,000 years.

The prophet Jeremiah condemns the cake-baking practice, saying it would provoke the one male god Yahweh to anger. But a later reference shows that people were determined to worship their goddess, the Queen of Heaven.

> Then all the men who knew that their wives were burning incense to other gods, along with all the women who were present – a large assembly – and all the people living in Lower and Upper Egypt, said to Jeremiah, 'We will not listen to the message you have spoken to us in the name of the LORD! We will certainly do everything we said we would: we will burn incense to the Queen of Heaven and will pour out drink offerings to her, just as we and our fathers, our kings and our officials did in the towns of Judah and in the streets of Jerusalem.

Incense, cakes, drink, girls' nights. I'm loving the sound of this!

Women aren't meekly bowing their heads to a male god here; it feels like something different entirely. You begin to get an inkling of what was stamped out by patriarchal Christianity, and it excites me.

But why am I discussing all this in a sex book? Well, because . . .

. . . when God is a woman it changes EVERYTHING. Especially sex.

This is not about believing in a God or Goddess, but

rather about glimpsing alternative realities which may have existed or could be possible. Irrespective of belief, we inherited a world where the all-powerful God has, for the last few thousand years, been worshipped as male, and it's been a time of subjugation for women's bodies, sexuality and spirituality. But if God is a woman, She has breasts, a vulva, a vagina. She grows, She ages, She bleeds. She goes through the menopause. She feels pleasure and pain. She has sex with who She wants, and She gives birth if She wants to and is able. She cannot be owned or violated because Her body is sacred.

Simply looking at the capitalisation of She, having been so used to the all-powerful He, shifts something for me, offering a flavour of a time when women weren't diminished. But the perhaps most exciting thing of all is to imagine an all-loving God of no gender and all genders – They or Them.

CURIOSITY

Answer the following questions in your journal.

How do you feel about the idea of God being a woman? What do you think about this?

How do you feel about the idea of God being of no gender?

What do you think about this?

SENSATION

Do your Before Care routine.

Yoni Massage

This is a massage of the vulva and vagina area. You will need some water-based lubricant.

I describe some strokes here that you might want to try, but do make this experience your own. Don't overthink it. Trust your intuition about what touch to give yourself. Always let the atmosphere and quality of touch be loving, reverent and curious.

Find a comfortable position, either lying on your back or sitting up with your legs open. Be as naked as you feel comfortable being. Start by doing the feather-like stroke touch up and down your whole body. Now, spend some time massaging the tops of your thighs in a circular motion in both directions.

Then gently rest your hands on top of your vulva, one on top of the other, and take some deep breaths with long, audible exhales. Spend some minutes here, slowly breathing in and out from the mouth and gently cupping your vulva. Allow your breaths to bring you to a sense of relaxation. Send love and tenderness to your vulva with your hands.

When you feel ready – and make sure your hands are well oiled – move your hands, one after the other, in upward strokes from your perineum to your mons pubis. Go slow, and breathe. Take pauses to rest and see how your body feels. Then change direction.

From the perineum, introduce some wide circular strokes, working round the whole of the outside of the vulva. Go slow, and breathe. Take pauses to rest and see how your body feels. Then change direction.

Then spend time slowly circling your clitoris. Go slow, and breathe. Take pauses to rest and see how your body feels. Then change direction.

Now spend time circling around the entrance to your vagina. Go slow, and breathe. Take pauses to rest and see how your body feels. Then change direction.

If you feel ready to, with whichever well-oiled finger(s) feels comfortable to you, start to tenderly and gently move your finger(s) inside your vagina. Using light pressure, work your way around, feeling the vaginal wall. Go slow, and breathe. Take pauses to rest and see how your body feels. Then change direction.

This exercise is about loving touch and massage for the vulva and vagina. It is not aimed at achieving orgasm or chasing a particular outcome. However, you might find that feelings of arousal or emotion wash over you as you do this exercise. Give these feelings the space to be. Breathe. Allow the experience to be what it will.

Finish the practice in whichever way feels nourishing for your body. You might feel the need to give yourself a hug, some self-pleasure, or to snuggle under a duvet.

After Care

Spend some time in stillness.

Be curious. Notice how you feel in your body.

Notice if any thoughts pop into your mind. Don't try to change anything. There is no right or wrong. Simply notice them.

Now journal on (or think about) the following questions:

How was that experience for me?
How am I feeling in this moment?
What do I need right now?

If you are able to, in a slow and mindful way, offer yourself some of what you need.

DEVOTION

Bake Sacred Vulva Cookies for the Queen of Heaven

On the next page is a recipe for the Jewish sweet treats called *hamantaschen*, which are eaten during the festival of Purim. Some Jewish commentators have noted that these traditional triangular pastries, filled with a poppyseed paste, may actually have been those baked in devotion to the goddess Ishtar[18] (who later became known as the Jewish heroine Esther when rabbis sought to erase the goddess and make the religion focus on one male god).

Could this recipe have survived for so long? It's wonderful to think that it has. The cookies certainly look like they could be symbols of a fertile, fruitful, sensual goddess.

---

18 https://www.heyalma.com/yes-theres-a-reason-hamantaschen-look-like-vaginas/

INGREDIENTS

For the dough

225g butter

100g sugar

1 egg

1 tsp vanilla

1 tsp lemon zest

1 tsp baking powder

Pinch of salt

275g flour

For the filling

100g freshly ground poppyseeds

80ml milk

30g butter

70g sugar

1 tbsp honey

Pinch of salt

Zest of half a lemon or orange

50g ground/finely chopped nuts (optional)

4 tbsp raisins (optional)

Icing sugar, for sprinkling on top (optional)

METHOD

For the dough
Preheat oven to 180°C/Gas Mark 5 and line a baking
    sheet with greaseproof paper.
Cream butter and sugar together.
Add the egg, vanilla, and the lemon zest, then mix
    well.
In a separate bowl, combine the baking powder, salt,
    and 250g of flour.
Mix together the wet and dry ingredients. The dough
    should not be sticky.
Wrap in clingfilm and refrigerate for at least 30 minutes.

For the filling
In a medium saucepan, place the poppyseeds, milk, butter, sugar, honey and salt. Cook over a medium-low heat,
stirring occasionally, for about ten minutes or until the
milk is absorbed and the mixture has thickened. Remove
from heat. Add the lemon/orange zest, nuts and raisins,
and mix together well. Let the filling cool to room tem-
perature before using.

When the dough is ready, sprinkle the work surface
with flour. Roll out the dough so that it is quite thin,
about the same height as a couple of 10p coins stacked
on top of each other.

Use a round cookie cutter (up to 10cm in diameter) to cut circles in the dough.

Place each circle of dough on the baking sheet.

Drop a teaspoon of filling onto each circle. Pinch the circle in three places to make a triangle. Use water if the dough isn't sticking.

Bake the cookies for 10–15 minutes at 180 degrees, until the edges start to go golden.

CREATIVITY

Create a piece of artwork that acknowledges, celebrates and honours your vulva. You could use words, images, music – whatever format or genre you feel drawn to.

YOUR INTIMACY

So far, we've been looking at and redefining the relationship we have with our bodies and genitals. In this section we turn our attention towards what's going on for us, sexually, at this stage in our lives. It's a bit like a sex-life audit.

DAY 14

I am sensation

If years of meditation haven't brought you bliss,
try masturbation instead . . . (not a joke).

Dara Shaa

How do we touch ourselves? Do we even touch ourselves? Ever? Properly?

I touch myself. These three words feel powerful put together, and tantalising. I was educated at a Catholic convent school, so touching myself there, between my legs, was forbidden. It was the kind of thing I would have had to confess to a priest.

I'm aware that you might be reading this with a slight smirk, thinking, 'But I'm just not that into touching myself. I don't do it, it's not my thing.' If so, I should warn you that it's my mission to change this, and have you revelling in the pleasure you can give yourself.

Some research studies have found that female masturbation can help fend off an early menopause[19] and ease chronic pain[20]. It increases body positivity[21] and decreases stress levels[22] – and let's not forget that it's pleasurable and fun. We are far more likely to orgasm during masturbation than with a partner.[23]

How we self-pleasure is going to vary hugely and look very different for all of us. Some readers will have a regular or frequent practice, while others will do so rarely, if at all. Some of us prefer to masturbate in bed, others in the shower or bath, and some in a forest under a full moon or at their desk while battling a deadline – you get the gist.

There will be readers who like to use their favourite sex toy – maybe a Rabbit, air tickler or massager wand. Others will happily make use of a showerhead or pillow. There will be people who like to read or watch erotic material to stimulate their sexual minds.

Our sexual fantasies, too, will be as wonderfully diverse

19 https://royalsocietypublishing.org/doi/10.1098/rsos.191020
20 https://www.jstor.org/stable/3812827
21 https://www.researchgate.net/publication/354089301_Masturbatory_Behavior_and_Body_Image_A_Study_Among_Brazilian_Women
22 https://www.medicalnewstoday.com/articles/masturbation-effects-on-brain#positive-effects
23 https://www.tandfonline.com/doi/abs/10.1080/0092623X .2019.1586021?journalCode=usmt20

as we are. There'll be an infinite variety of playing and shapeshifting going on in our minds. Different partners, famous partners, numerous partners, on a beach, in a five-star hotel, in space! We might revel in being submissive, being taken forcibly or being teased for hours, or we may be the dominant one. Our sexual minds delight in us stating our desires.

Now, let's have a look at our self-pleasure scripts and see how they are working for us.

CURIOSITY

To start

Answer the following question in your journal.

What messages did you learn about self-pleasure when you were growing up?

Main exercise

Answer the following questions about your experiences of self-pleasure.

What tends to prompt you wanting to offer yourself some self-pleasure?

Where do you generally do it?

How do you prepare for it?

Do you use any erotic aids (e.g. sex toys, porn, etc.)? If so, what are they and why do you use them?

How do you usually begin?

Where and how do you touch yourself?

What might you be thinking during your self-pleasure session?

Do you have fantasies? If so, what are they? (We will be exploring fantasies in more detail on Day 20.)

What do you particularly enjoy about the experience?

Do you experience orgasm(s)/climax(es)?

If so, what normally prompts this climactic state?

And what does this climactic state feel like?

What do you do at the end of your self-pleasure session?

How do you feel afterwards?

What is it like to think about and write all this?

Do you have any thoughts about your self-pleasure practice now?

SENSATION

Give yourself a self-pleasure session exactly as you would normally. Afterwards, take some time to think about the experience. How do you feel now? What words might you use to describe your self-pleasure session? What words would you like to use about your self-pleasure sessions? Is there anything you would want to change or experiment with next time you self-pleasure?

DAY 15

I am connection

I don't identify as a woman, but I identify with
womanhood. Sex holds a lot of significance for me,
and I'm sure it does for other trans people. We are
sharing our bodies with someone else in such an intimate
way, it's an emotional space. It's one of the only spaces
where I feel like I am seen as I am.

Cal, England

In partnered sex, two or more people get together with
their own brand of beautifully fucked-up perfection to
share their bodies and experience sensations together. The
result can be anything from blissful and transcendent to
painful and traumatic, via a fair bit of OK, all right and a
bit meh.

For some readers, sex with another person will be a memory from years ago; others may be lying post-coital with a partner as they read this. Some people will have one regular partner; others may have many. Our lovers will be from different nationalities, cultures, heritages, classes. They might have a disability, whether mental or physical. They might be robust or frail, in chronic pain, ill or undergoing medical treatment. They will range in age, personality and temperament. Some will be living, as Instagram says, 'their best life', while others will be facing personal challenges. For some, sex is where they are at their most confident; for others, sex is where they feel at their most vulnerable.

But what do we do with these people? We are going to have a little look at what goes on when we are sexual with others, by noticing the process and paying particular attention to our thoughts and feelings about it. Sex scripts can get tired and staid, cluttered with bits we're not that fond of, but do anyway. This exercise can act like a spring clean, whether or not we are currently having partnered sex.

CURIOSITY

To start

Answer the following question in your journal.

What did you learn about partnered sexual experiences when you were growing up?

Main exercise

Answer the following questions about your partnered sexual experiences.

What normally prompts sexual activity to take place?
Who instigates, and how? (How does this make you feel? Do any thoughts go through your head about this?)
How does the sexual activity start?
Is there kissing? (How does this make you feel? Do any thoughts go through your head about this?)
Does your partner touch your body? If so, where and how? (How does this feel? Do any thoughts go through your head about this?)

Do you touch your partner's body? If so, where and how? (How does this feel? Do any thoughts go through your head about this?)

Does there tend to be a progression of activities? If so, what is the progression? Who instigates the start of each new activity, and how? (How does this feel? Do any thoughts go through your head about this?)

Is there penetration of the mouth, vagina, anus? (How does this feel? Do any thoughts go through your head about this?)

Do you reach a climactic state of pleasure, or orgasm? If so, when does this occur? What prompts it? (How does it feel? Do any thoughts go through your head about this?)

How do you feel afterwards?

What are the highlights of this experience for you?

Which are the parts you least enjoy?

What does it feel like to think about all this? What thoughts or feelings do you now have about your partnered sexual experiences?

SENSATION

Solo Practice

Recall an instance of partnered sex and follow the path it took as a template for a self-pleasure session. For example, if it started with you lying on your side, kissing your partner, lie on your side and touch your lips and tongue. Then continue to touch yourself where you were touched, and move your body into the positions you were in while with your partner.

Afterwards, notice how this experience was for you.

Were there any full heart yes moments in the experience for you? Do you have any thoughts about your partnered sex sessions now? Do you have any thoughts about your self-pleasure sessions now?

Partnered Practice (optional)

If you have a sexual partner, then then you might want to experience some sexual activity with them. Afterwards, take some time to think about the experience.

How do you feel now in your body? Were there any full heart yes moments in the experience for you? What words might you use to describe your partnered sexual experience? What words would you like to use about your partnered sexual experience? Is there anything you would want to change, or experiment with, next time you experience partnered sex?

YOUR PLEASURE

In this part of the book, we explore sexual arousal. How does it feel? Where does it move? What activates it – and deactivates it?

DAY 16

I am arousal

When I first started exploring my body, I didn't really know what was possible, but I understood that getting to know myself for pleasure was an act of rebellion.

Nimko Ali

We'll be spending the next few days looking at what arouses us and brings us sexual pleasure. Consider this your personal pleasure school, where you have full permission to find out what you like. If you haven't done this before, I hope it marks the start of a love of learning in this area.

We can become aroused in a variety of ways, but today we'll focus on where you like to be touched, and how you like this touch to be. Studies have reliably shown that women have a greater variety of erogenous zones than men, with the most powerful being breasts and nipples, lips, neck, nape of neck, ears and buttocks. One study cited that 12% of women could achieve orgasm through the stimulation of these areas alone.[24]

These are by no means all the areas of the body that might feel good to be touched. You might love behind your knee, the inside of your wrist, your armpit, your lower belly, inner thighs or scalp being touched, for instance.

But instead of reading studies and articles that tell us which areas of the female body are sensitive or pleasurable to touch, we're going to find out what works for us.

CURIOSITY

Read the following, then write about it in your journal.

Recall a time when you very much enjoyed being touched. This could be touch you received from someone else or touch that you gave yourself. Write about this experience.

---

24 https://journals.lww.com/humanandrology/Abstract/2016/03000/ Female_hot_spots__extragenital_erogenous_zones.4.aspx

Some things to consider: Where were you? Where were you touched? What was the quality of the touch? What words would you use to describe the experience? Why does this experience stand out from others?

In your journal, draw an outline of your body. This is for you to use after the next exercise.

SENSATION

Touching your Body

Do your Before Care routine. Imagine you are a sensual lover, discovering your own body for the first time. You are going to cover your body, including all nooks and crannies, in a variety of touches to discover your sensitive and pleasurable spots.

I have added some pointers here, but when it comes to discovering the touch you like, feel free to throw the book on the floor, use your intuition and freestyle!

You might like to have some massage oil available. Before you begin, here are some types of touch you might like to try:

- a light touch, using the fingertips.
- a light scratch, using fingernails.
- holding an area firmly.
- long, firm, gliding strokes.
- a rhythmic touch (i.e., find a rhythm for a particular touch and stay with it for a while)
- any other touch you feel drawn to.

Now, take each of the below areas in turn and spend time touching them thoroughly.

- head, scalp and ears
- face, including mouth and tongue
- neck, collarbone and shoulders
- arms and hands
- chest and breasts
- as much of your back as you can reach!
- belly and waist
- thighs and bottom
- legs
- feet.

(This is not necessarily a genital touch exercise, but of course if you would like to include the genitals in this exercise, please do.)

The main thing to remember? *Don't rush!* Allow enough time on each area and with each type of touch. Touch an area for a while, then stop, breathe, and notice how you are feeling before trying a new touch or area.

Afterwards, decorate the sketch of your body you drew earlier to show how your body responds to touch. Highlight your sensitive areas in whichever way you wish. Feel free to get creative: you could use paint, glitter, stickers, colours, collage, words or anything else that inspires you.

You might even like to draw some more sketches, focusing on particular body parts and their sensitivity. You may also like to revisit this exercise at a later date to see if your 'body touch map' has changed at all.

After Care

Spend some time in stillness.

Be curious. Notice how you feel in your body.

Notice if any thoughts pop into your mind. Don't try to change anything. There is no right or wrong. Simply notice them.

Now journal on (or think about) the following questions:

How was that experience for me?
How am I feeling in this moment?
What do I need right now?

If you are able to, in a slow and mindful way, offer yourself some of what you need.

DAY 17

I am activation

In my family, sex was always a taboo, never talked about.
Questions weren't allowed; it's like you were supposed to
be born knowing everything.

Monica, Spain

The female genitals are so densely packed with nerve endings that you'd think we'd be able to give them a quick fondle
and *boom* – we'd be aroused. But for most of us, that isn't
the case. If I stroke my genitals now I'll feel pretty much
nothing, even if I rub them for a while. It seems as though
my genitals need to be activated before they can be touched
directly, and I've discovered that there are a lot of stimuli,
both physical and mental, that can activate them.

Diana Richardson in her book, *The Heart of Tantric Sex,*

explains that sexual energy moves in our bodies from a positive pole to a negative pole, a bit like a battery. The positive pole must be stimulated before the negative pole can become activated. In bodies with penises, the penis is the positive pole and the negative pole is the chest and heart area. However, this is not the case in bodies with vulvas. Here the vulva and vagina are considered to constitute the negative pole, with the positive pole being the chest and heart area. According to this school of thought, you would need to pay attention to the upper body, in particular the heart and breast area, to activate the genitals.

Katinka Soetens, my sacred sexual priestess teacher, goes even further. She maintains that female external genitals can be viewed as comprising two opposing poles, with the upper part of the genitals being the positive and the lower the negative. In this framework the clitoral glans and upper parts of the labia are stimulated to activate the lower genitals and the entrance to the vagina. I find these sexuality teachings illuminating to explore, and they often feel very true in my body.

But we are all different, and arousal won't feel the same for everyone. It will come in different places and paces. It is even unlikely to stay the same for us throughout our lives; rather, it alters as we journey through life and womanhood.

DAY 17

CURIOSITY

Answer the following questions in your journal.

Think of a time when you experienced great sexual pleasure. Can you see where and how sexual arousal was activated and moved in your body?
Now think of a time when you had a sexual experience that wasn't so satisfying. Can you see how and where sexual energy didn't move in your body?

SENSATION

Explore whether upper body and breast/chest stimulation arouses your genitals

Do your Before Care routine. Lie down naked or in as few clothes as possible. Spend five minutes doing the Light Activation Meditation (see p. 31). Set a timer for fifteen minutes. You may well resist this and think it feels like

151

an incredibly long time. Sadly, this is natural in today's fast-paced world, which doesn't prioritise pleasure. But let's be radical: let's define ourselves as Pleasure Seekers, as Ridwana Jooma, Johannesburg-based sexuality coach and one of my inspirations, calls us.

Spend fifteen minutes stimulating the upper body, chest and breasts. Relax into the time allowed here, start slowly and breathe. Follow your intuition, using whatever touch feels good. Take time to touch, stroke and massage your breasts before you begin to touch your nipples. Afterwards, do you feel any sexual activation in your genitals? Do you feel that your genitals would enjoy being touched now? (If so, carry on to the next part below.)

Explore whether stimulation of the upper vulva activates the vagina

Spend fifteen minutes touching your genitals. Again, relax into the time allowed here, start slowly and breathe. Spend time exploring, touching and stroking the upper parts of your vulva, including circling and touching the clitoris.

Then explore touching around and in the entrance to your vagina.

Did you learn anything today about arousal and how it moves in your body? Does the notion of positive and negative poles feel true to your body?

After Care

Spend some time in stillness.

Be curious. Notice how you feel in your body.

Notice if any thoughts pop into your mind. Don't try to change anything. There is no right or wrong. Simply notice them.

Now journal on (or think about) the following questions:

How was that experience for me?
How am I feeling in this moment?
What do I need right now?

If you are able to, in a slow and mindful way, offer yourself some of what you need.

CREATIVITY

If you enjoyed decorating the sketch of your body on Day 16, you might like to draw an outline of your body again – and your vulva. Then draw, write on, colour or decorate them to show how sexual arousal moves around your body.

DAY 18

I am excitement

My husband is turned on by me dressing up in the beautiful, ridiculously skimpy, sexy underwear he buys me. It's kind of fun for me, but it won't turn me on. I thought, 'What do I need?' And the answer was heaps of talking. I want to know what's going on in his mind.

Kate, New Zealand

There is, of course, one rather important erogenous zone we haven't yet mentioned: the brain. It isn't just touching our body that activates arousal: it can also be stimulating material such as watching people be sexual on screen, reading an erotic story, looking at the human body or hearing a husky voice telling us to hold during a phone call. Research shows that for some people, just thinking about their nipples and genitals being touched sexually can lead to arousal or even orgasm.[25]

However, there's more at play than simply putting erotic content in our path and feeling arousal. The human brain comprises a rather cool-sounding mechanism called the Sexual Excitation System (SES).[26] The SES notices all our turn-ons, so in order for us to be sexually aroused it has to be switched on – and kept on. It sounds very simple, and it is, although admittedly it becomes a little more problematic when we discover that there is also a Sexual Inhibition System, which effectively serves as a fire blanket over this excitement.

Emily Nagoski, author of the fantastic book *Come As You Are*, refers to all the things that turn on our Sexual Excitation System as our *accelerators*. They are all the things that are sexually relevant to us, and allow us to feel open to arousal. These can range from having a tidy bedroom and a completed to-do list, to words of appreciation and love, to being spanked on the bottom with a paddle.

25 https://www.ncbi.nlm.nih.gov/pmc/articles/PMC5084724/#CIT0033
26 https://kinseyinstitute.org/pdf/Factoranalysis.pdf

CURIOSITY

In your journal, make a list of your sexual accelerators: all the things that help you feel arousal and excitement. To do this, it might help if you thought of all the ways you could finish this sentence:

It is possible for me to get sexually excited when . . .

We want a really big long list that you can keep adding to, so consider the following, adding as many items as you can:

My physical well-being, e.g. when I have taken my pain medication.

My appearance, e.g. when I have shaved my legs.

My environment e.g. when the house is quiet and tidy.

What has gone on beforehand, e.g. when I have had a bath and had time to relax after putting the kids to bed.

My relationship, e.g. when my partner and I have spent some time chatting and connecting together beforehand.

Erotic stimuli, e.g. when I watch porn that shows . . .

Sexual activities and techniques, e.g. when I do lots of sensual kissing.

Anything else I can think of.

Afterwards, look at your list. Does it surprise you in any way? Is there anything you can take from this exercise that will be useful?

SENSATION

Think Yourself Off

Do your Before Care routine. From this relaxed place, think about all your accelerators. Spend at least ten minutes very slowly imagining a scenario where you are experiencing many of your accelerators. Give these imaginings as much detail and colour as possible in your mind.

Now imagine yourself receiving, from yourself or another person, touch to your erogenous areas. If you think you can orgasm in this way, go ahead – but, as ever, there is absolutely no pressure on you to feel anything here. We are simply being curious about whether we can activate arousal through thought alone.

End, as usual, with After Care.

DAY 19

I am discernment

Smell, for me, is the biggest turn-on or -off. Often, I'll see the client through the intercom camera as I let them in. They look young and good-looking, and I think, 'Sweet', but they don't smell nice so it's hard work. But if they smell nice I can get super turned-on.

Dani, Australia

But what about our turn-*offs*?

As I mentioned in Day 18, running in parallel with our Sexual Excitation System is our Sexual Inhibition System. This is everything that *stops* our excitement and shuts down our capacity for arousal. Emily Nagoski refers to this as our brakes. Our brakes may be very sensitive, and many things will activate them, including certain sights and smells, words and actions, distractions and disturbances.

I remember once a chap I was with used the word 'tits' in bed. He'd been paying attention to and touching my breasts, which is a big accelerator for me, and had said something complimentary about my breasts, which again is an accelerator, but the word 'tits' put an emergency stop to my arousal. All I could think about from then on was how much I hated that word. My sister had a similar experience when a lover she was with started sniffing her pants after she had taken them off.

Many of our brakes will feel more subtle than this, though. Netflix puts my brakes on. If after dinner I sit on the sofa and start watching an American serialised drama, it will take a *lot* of accelerators to get me feeling aroused afterwards.

CURIOSITY

In your journal, write as many responses as you can to the following:

I am not open to sexual excitement when . . .
I get turned off when . . .

SENSATION

Breathgasms

Throughout this book, we have been noticing and exploring the breath. We have been allowing our deep, long, audible breaths to calm and centre us. Today I invite you to use your breath in a more dynamic way, to potentially access an ecstatic state. Nowadays there is a lot of discussion about breathwork. You may have come across the Wim Hof Method®, tantric breathing, holotropic breathwork or perhaps Barbara Carrellas's breath and energy orgasm.

Most dynamic breathing practices follow a similar structure: a period of dynamic, audible circular breathing (i.e. with no gap between inhale and exhale), followed by some sort of breath hold or squeeze. Visualisation may also be used to intensify the experience.

Do the following practice as often as you desire.

If it appeals to you, allow yourself to discover your own practice in this sphere. Search on the internet for different breath practices and try them out. Have a go at playing with the elements of circular breathing, visualisation and movement, and with the intensity you bring to it. You might think, I'll spend 5 minutes breathing deeply and imagining myself being filled with joy or playfulness or confidence, then I'll hold the breath for a while and when I release the breath I'll send all my joy out into the world. Have fun with your breath, your imagination, your body. Find what feels good and nourishing for you. Be curious and see what happens.

Take time to read through the exercise a few times before you begin.

100 Breaths to Ecstasy

I love the beautiful simplicity of this practice. My dear friend Simon Paul Sutton showed it to me, and it is a practice he teaches in his self-pleasure courses.

100 Breaths to Ecstasy will gently train your body to get used to a deeper breath frequency and absorb more oxygen. Deep breathing is believed to have many benefits: it has been found to improve anxiety, depression and post-traumatic stress disorder (PTSD), increase pain thresholds, reduce blood pressure and heart rate, and strengthen the lungs and diaphragm.[27]

I regularly do this as a standalone practice to shift my mood and energy level when I'm feeling down or

---

27 https://www.ncbi.nlm.nih.gov/pmc/articles/PMC5455070/

sluggish. I also love it as a precursor to self-pleasure and partnered sex.

Do your Before Care routine. Sit on a chair with your feet flat on the floor, or cross-legged. Keep your arms relaxed and your back straight. Your posture should be wide and open.

Take the time to slow down and breathe. Give your hips a wiggle, and rock back and forth on your seat bones until you find the perfect position. Now shift your awareness to your head and neck. Let your head drop gently forward so your chin points towards your chest, then drop your head back so your chin points towards the sky. Be very gentle here and only drop your head to where it feels comfortable. Do this a few times, then find the balance spot where your head rests comfortably on your neck.

Relax your mouth, have a big yawn, stretch your mouth in all directions. Feel how beautiful it is to release all the tension in your jaw. As it's so beautiful, do it one more time. Then come to rest with your mouth open.

Breathe in and out through your open mouth. Emphasise the inhale, and let go on the exhale. Try some practice breaths now. Find a rhythm where your breathing becomes circular and there are no gaps or pauses.

Place your hands on your belly and heart so you can track your breath. On an inhale your belly and chest will expand; on an exhale they will fall. Open your mouth wide to allow the breath to come in and flow out. Take 100 breaths in this way. Allow the breath to do its magic. If you find your mind wandering during the 100 breaths, don't worry; simply bring your mind back to the breathing.

Emotions may rise. When we breathe deeply, we can take the lid off any suppressed emotions. If that happens, allow them as fully as you can. If they seem to be overwhelming, simply open your eyes and come back to the moment. You may feel pins and needles or a tingling sensation all over your body. This is normal and natural. Just observe it.

Taking the 100 breaths takes about five minutes. If you lose count, don't worry – just pick up from the last number you remember. On the last exhale, gently release your breath and explore the sweet place there between the breaths.

When you feel the impulse to inhale, do so. Take life in. Then return to normal breathing.

Spend some time with your eyes closed. When you are ready to, open your eyes. Observe how you feel. End, as usual, with After Care.

DAY 20

I am fantasy

I have no idea why that ended up in my library of fantasies.

Jessica, Canada

We'll now turn our attention to the fantasy scripts that play out in our minds and ignite our arousal. For some of us, our fantasies will be like a prized film collection which we enjoy choosing from during lovemaking and self-pleasure. 'Hmm, shall I be the queen or the subject today? Shall we be in the palace or the garden?' But for others, our fantasies may feel more like a crutch – something we can't give up. We use them, feeling ashamed, and afterwards wish we hadn't.

Our fantasies are a bit like our sexual dream-state. They emanate from our subconscious, so we're not always able to control them.

It's important to know that, however weird we think our fantasies might be, we are *normal*. Research shows that that there are hardly any rare or statistically unusual sexual fantasies, and that what people tend to fantasise about is not necessarily what they are interested in doing in person.[28]

Jack Morin, in his famous book *The Erotic Mind*, discusses how we all have a 'core erotic theme' – a fantasy that will always turn us on. When we look at it, this can often be traced back to an emotional state we felt when we were young. It can be insightful to take some time to think about our fantasies – and how and why they may have originated.

CURIOSITY

Take some time to explore the following questions in your journal.

What were your first sexual fantasies?
What was the last sexual fantasy you had?
How do you feel about having sexual fantasies?
How have your sexual fantasies changed throughout your life?

---

28 https://www.sciencedirect.com/science/article/pii/S2352250X22002172

Can you spot the key themes or characteristics in your fantasies?

Can you spot how and why these themes and characteristics materialised?

Are there any aspects of your fantasies that you would like to bring into your lived experience?

SENSATION

Self-pleasure with Fantasy

Do your Before Care routine. Sit or lie down. Establish a relaxed breathing rhythm with bigger than normal inhales and longer audible exhales.

When you have established this breathing rhythm, introduce a gentle rocking of the hips. If it works for you to do so, then exhale as your hips go back and inhale as they go forward. When the hips are in this forward position lightly clench and squeeze the pelvic floor and bottom muscles.

Play with the pace and intensity of this combination of movement and audible breath for some time. Notice how it feels in your body.

When you are ready to, engage with your erotic mind and visualise or feel into a fantasy of your choosing. What sort of fantasy are you drawn to today?

Don't rush. Take the time to add details and embellishment to your fantasy. Allow yourself to enjoy it. Create your own fantastic sensual feast in your mind. Feel free to touch your body as you wish.

After Care

Spend some time in stillness.

Be curious. Notice how you feel in your body.

Notice if any thoughts pop into your mind. Don't try to change anything. There is no right or wrong. Simply notice them.

Now journal on (or think about) the following questions:

How was that experience for me?
How am I feeling in this moment?
What do I need right now?

If you are able to, in a slow and mindful way, offer yourself some of what you need.

DAY 21

I am eroticism

Ban it? Feminism doesn't need to start BANNING pornography. It needs to start MAKING it.

Caitlin Moran

Pornography is content of a sexual nature designed to stir sensations of arousal in the body and awaken the erotic mind.

I'm going to refer to pornography as erotic content from now on. This is because online porn is so prevalent nowadays that it might be all we think of when we talk about pornography. But that excludes a plethora of other erotic content, such as art, literature, graphic novels, photography, audio recordings, music and just about any other creative art form you can think of.

There will be content out there that arouses us – we may not have found it yet. And that which arouses us might not even show genitals, or touching. It might not fall easily under the 'pornography' banner; it might be far more subtle, involving sounds or suggestions.

When I interviewed women for my book *Women on Top of the World*, I was struck by the variety and creativity of the erotic content that aroused women, from ASMR (autonomous sensory meridian response) audio recordings of voices saying, 'Hey, babe, are you home?' to erotic cartoons of wizards.

What arouses *you*? And how comfortable and at home do you feel here in the realm of pornography and erotica?

CURIOSITY

Answer the following question in your journal.

What erotic content have you consumed in your life?

Which elements or parts of this erotic content have aroused you? What words would you use to describe the erotic content you have consumed? What words would you like to use to describe the erotic content available to you?

SENSATION

Self-pleasure with Erotic Content

Do your Before Care routine. Allow yourself to look for and find something you enjoy and find arousing or potentially arousing. This could be art, movie, porn clips, audio recordings, stories, etc.

You might use some of your key words from the Curiosity section above to help with your search. Spend 15–20 minutes exploring erotic content. Enjoy touching your body too, if that feels good.

After Care

Spend some time in stillness.

Be curious. Notice how you feel in your body.

Notice if any thoughts pop into your mind. Don't try to change anything. There is no right or wrong. Simply notice them.

Now journal on (or think about) the following questions:

How was that experience for me?
How am I feeling in this moment?
What do I need right now?

If you are able to, in a slow and mindful way, offer yourself some of what you need.

CREATIVITY

Create a work of erotic content: it could be a story, photograph, piece of artwork, collage, audio recording, anything! Create it with the aim of gently (or rigorously) arousing *you*.

YOUR DESIRE

This is where the magic is!

DAY 22

I am desire

My mum is a priestess of Isis. She taught me to stand under the full moon, to inhale its power, feel it seep into my being. Then to slowly say, 'I refuse to accept anything less than everything I desire.'

Priestess Bliss Magdalena

This might be the most important day of all.

As women, when it comes to sex, we often know what we *don't* like but we aren't so sure about what we actually *do* want. This tends to be simply because we've never thought about what *we* desire when it comes to sex, or felt able to ask ourselves this question.

Perhaps the simplest and most profound words we can whisper to ourselves when it comes to sexuality are, 'What do I want?' As Jaya from Ecuador says, it 'is one of the scariest and most freeing questions'. We shouldn't underestimate how life-changing (and world-changing) this one question can be.

Sexual energy is life energy. Saying yes to pleasure, to connection, to sensation, to experience, to desire, to *yourself*, means saying YES to LIFE, and the effects will reverberate throughout all facets of your existence.

CURIOSITY

To start

Answer the following question in your journal.

In your everyday life, how connected are you to your desires?

Main exercise

Write a list of everything you'd like to experience in your sexual life. Think about your list, then write a list of words that describe how you want to feel during these experiences.

SENSATION

Sex Magic Ritual

Perform sex magic to manifest your desires! You can go to town on this exercise or do it in a more low-key way – just find the way that suits you. The aim is to create a ritual to wish your dreams well, to super-charge them with sexual energy, then send them out into the world to be made real.

Ensure that nothing on your sexual desires list could harm anyone else, and that your dreams are for the highest good for all.

Consider when you might like to do this practice.

Before Care

Create a circle on the floor, the bed or the ground around you. You could mark this out with chalk, or with scarves, wool, etc. Inside, you might like to add some objects that feel symbolic to you and your dreams.

Write your desires or some of your key words on a piece of paper, card, stone, or other object. Decorate this with any symbols that feel meaningful. Feel free to decorate your body, too, with any words and symbols that feel meaningful to your desires.

Create an intentional or sacred space in whichever way feels right for you. You may like to sing a devotional song, or say a prayer or poem. You could simply repeat the affirmation from the beginning of this chapter: 'I refuse to accept anything less than *everything* I desire.'

Start by dancing or doing the Light Activation Meditation or another practice to make you feel connected to yourself and open to all that is. Say your desires aloud as you hold your object or paper. Then lay the object or paper either in between your legs or nearby.

Give yourself a self-pleasure session. Take time during the session to imagine your dreams coming true. Imagine that your sexual energy is charging up your dreams and bringing them to life. As you reach a climax, imagine all your orgasmic energy being channelled into your beautiful dreams. As you rest afterwards, take some moments to send some love and perhaps a smile to others who might also be doing, or have carried out, this ritual.

May all your dreams come true.

After Care

Spend some time in stillness.

Be curious. Notice how you feel in your body.

Notice if any thoughts pop into your mind. Don't try to change anything. There is no right or wrong. Simply notice them.

Now journal on (or think about) the following questions:

How was that experience for me?
How am I feeling in this moment?
What do I need right now?

If you are able to, in a slow and mindful way, offer yourself some of what you need.

YOUR POWER

In this part we look at our ability to voice our wants and wishes, and how we say yes and no. We wonder too about the power dynamics that exist in our sexual connections: we look at what they are and what they could be.

DAY 23

I am yes and I am no

For me to say these things was unprecedented.
I remember shaking, my voice trembling, but it was
probably the bravest thing I've done in my personal life.
I am so glad I did it, because he told me about this weird
sexual thing that he had going on too.

Olga, Russia

I'm going to share a memory now which saddens me every time I think about it. One year at Glastonbury Festival I went to a talk about Taoist sexuality. A man gave the talk. He seemed quite nice – he spoke about how sex could be slow and mindful, which I liked. At one point a young man raised his hand to ask a question. His girlfriend was leaning against him, her head nestled into his shoulder.

'But is it OK to do hard fucking?' the young man asked.

The teacher looked at him, gave a smile and a small chuckle. 'Yes.' He nodded.

None of the women present said anything at all about how 'hard fucking' might feel for us. Clearly, neither of the men thought to ask us how we felt about 'hard fucking'. The men laughed as they discussed what it was OK to do to our bodies, and the women sat silent. I often think about that day and I wish I could rewind time. There is so much I could say about 'hard fucking', and about when it feels great – and when it most definitely doesn't.

I don't think we should ever underestimate how difficult it is for many women to speak up about our experience of sex, either in the moment or later. To say 'no' or 'that's too much for me' or 'I'm not ready for that right now' or 'that hurts'.

The sex festivals I have been to have all started with workshops where attendees are given time to practise asking for what they want, and saying and hearing the word 'yes' – and, more crucially, the word 'no'.

Tantra teacher and relationship expert Jan Day holds workshops all over the world for people to explore intimacy and sexuality. She says, 'We have to learn that it is totally fine for anyone to want anything, and also that it's totally fine to say no. It's OK to *not* get, and it is OK to *not* give. Both are OK.'

We need to practise connecting with, and voicing, our

whole-hearted 'YES' and our absolute 'NO', and to discover that we are OK after saying either.

CURIOSITY

Answer the following question in your journal.

How good are you at saying no in your life?

Think about all areas of your life: your work life, your family life, your sex life. Do you ever say yes when you would like to say no, or vice versa? And how whole-hearted are you when you say yes?

SENSATION

The Bossy Massage

Give and receive a bossy massage with a friend or lover. This is a great way to practise giving and receiving feedback regarding touch and sex.

Take some Before Care time with your partner. Here, you should discuss place, practicalities and boundaries. Where will you position yourselves? Will you be sitting or lying down? Are you warm enough?

You should both state your boundaries beforehand and come to a comfortable agreement. Will you be clothed, partially clothed or naked? What areas of the body are out of bounds? Who will be asking the questions first?

Now think in terms of mind, body and spirit – is there anything you might like to do to help you feel more connected to yourselves and each other before you start? This could be meditation, eye gazing, each taking a minute to say how you are feeling, sharing loving words, shaking or dancing.

The Boss is the person receiving the massage. The Toucher, as the name suggests, is the person giving the touch. The Boss is completely in charge. They get to tell the Toucher exactly where and how they want to be massaged and touched, while the Toucher does only what the Boss says – and of course this includes saying 'no' if they are not comfortable with what they are being asked to do.

Set the timer for five minutes. Get bossing!

Set the timer for another three minutes and spend some time talking about how the exercise was for you. How did it feel to give and receive instruction? What did you like and dislike?

Then swap roles and repeat.

Remember: When you are the Boss, experiment with how you can ask for what you want: for example, 'Please can you . . .', 'I'd like it like . . .', 'Touch me there', 'Here! Now!' or 'Firmer!' You can exaggerate your role and be playful with it.

As the Toucher, if you're not given an instruction, don't do anything. Wait to be told. Don't freestyle or intuit what the Boss wants.

Afterwards, spend some After Care time with your partner. Share any final thoughts about the practice, what you learned, etc. Thank each other. See if there might be a nice way for you to end your time together – a hug? Cup of tea? Sandwich?

DAY 24

I am dominance and I am submission

I am not submissive to everybody, but I am submissive to those who know how to appreciate my submissiveness. The devotion of a woman or man is a very special gift.

Anja, Germany

Consensual sex can be a glorious playground for power.

We can feel the intensity of submissiveness as we hang on every word and touch from a masterful lover, or we can experience the thrill of taking control of the action, demanding that we be worshipped in the exact way we wish. Perhaps we switch between the two. Playing with power dynamics in a clear way can be thrilling.

Those who engage in dominance and submission play have reported psychological benefits similar to those associated with meditation, hobbies and sport: better concentration, less mental activity, better ability to live 'in the moment', relaxation and increased feelings of well-being. Conscious play with dominance and submission focuses our attention in a manner akin to mindfulness.

But there may be power dynamics in our sexual lives that we haven't consciously chosen, and these can feel more complicated, blurry or unsatisfying. We might feel that we are playing a role that is expected of us, but that we don't really fit. Perhaps we long to be more dominant, but feel we should be nice, polite, submissive. Or maybe we're tired of always initiating and driving sex and long to feel the power and passion of a dominant other.

In long-term relationships we can easily get stuck in sex scripts and power dynamics that stopped working for us long ago. I think it is interesting to note that research has shown that our preference for power roles tends not to stay static over time.[29]

So how do you feel about your own experience of dominance and submission? Have you explored all you wish to in this area, or are there elements you feel would be interesting or arousing to try? Do you feel able to play with power roles, or do you feel that one power role has been thrust upon you?

---

29 https://www.tandfonline.com/doi/full/10.1080/00224499.2020.1767025

CURIOSITY

To start

Answer the following question in your journal.

When do you feel powerful in your life?
When do you feel submissive in your life?

Main exercise

Answer the following question in your journal.

What sexual power role(s) do you tend to play?

In partnered sexual experiences, do you tend to hold a position of power over the other person, or vice versa? And if so, is this a conscious decision taken by you both, or not? Are you happy with the power dynamics in your partnered sexual experiences? If so, why? And if not, why not? What sexual power roles would you like to play?

SENSATION

The Three-Minute Game
(to be played with a friend or lover)

This game was devised by Harry Faddis as part of a BDSM (bondage and discipline, domination and submission) workshop in New York. You will find a lot of information online about the Three-Minute Game – Betty Martin, who we met earlier when we did the Waking Up the Hands exercise, in particular, is a big advocate of it.

The game is delightfully simple but hugely powerful. Play it with a partner, either sexual or platonic. Take some Before Care time with your partner. As before, you can discuss place, practicalities and boundaries. Where will you position yourselves? Will you be sitting or lying down? Are you warm enough?

You should state your boundaries beforehand and come to an agreement. Will you be clothed, partially clothed or naked? What areas of the body are out of bounds? Who will be asking the questions first?

Now think in terms of mind, body and spirit – is there anything you might like to do to help you feel more connected to yourselves and each other before you start? You might consider meditating, eye gazing, each having a minute to say how you are feeling, sharing loving words, shaking or dancing.

When you are both ready . . .

Person 1 asks, 'How do you want me to touch you for three minutes?'

Person 2 explains the touch they would like to receive. After they have stated a desire, the two can still negotiate until they reach agreement. Both must be comfortable with what is about to happen.

Set the timer for three minutes.

For three minutes, Person 1 gives Person 2 the touch they desire.

Person 2 has to describe what they want, so that they receive the experience they want.

Person 1 asks, 'How do you want to touch me for three minutes?'

Person 2 explains how they would like to touch Person 1. They reach an agreement. Then Person 1 allows Person 2 to touch their body. This is for the pleasure of Person 2 rather than Person 1 (although they too might enjoy it). Person 1 must say 'Stop' or 'No' if they are uncomfortable with the touch they are being given.

Then swap roles and repeat.

Afterwards, spend some After Care time with your partner. Set the timer for another three minutes and talk about how the exercise was for you. How did it feel to give and receive instruction? What did you both like and dislike? What did you learn? Thank each other. See if there might be a nice way for you to end your time together: a hug? A cup of tea? Sandwich?

YOUR PLAYFULNESS

In this part of the book we cultivate an attitude of joy, lightness and exploration in our sexuality. I wonder what would happen if . . . ?

DAY 25

I am playfulness

I like to be really free and very playful while I'm having sex: I like to play music and take a lot of pictures. I am very visual. I like to wear robes and try out toys, just kind of messing.

Linda, Czech Republic

Of all the interviews I have conducted and the conversations I have had with women about their sexual experiences, I have heard the word 'playful' used only a handful of times. I can't help giving a little gasp of delight when it pops up in conversation. Somehow this word, more than any other, conjures a sense of lightness and joy around sexuality. Sadly, I very infrequently hear it used by women in heterosexual relationships.

One definition of playfulness is the way people 'frame or reframe everyday situations in a way such that they experience them as entertaining, and/or intellectually stimulating, and/or personally interesting'.[30]

The thought that I most associate with playfulness is 'I wonder what might happen if . . .' It feels so pregnant with possibilities, and devoid of fear or shame.

'I wonder what might happen if I lick her there.'

'I wonder what would happen if I tease them by sending them this erotic message.'

'I wonder what might happen if I suggest some naked wrestling.'

My buddy Neil Morbey (irreverent fool, mindfulness coach and pleasure hound as he (playfully) describes himself) loves an acronym. He says that PLAY could stand for Pure Living Allowing You. I love that.

Studies have shown that being more playful has positive outcomes across all areas of life, and recent research[31] shows that adults can cultivate playfulness even if they are very serious. Contrary to what you might expect, becoming more playful, the study found, can be relatively easy. In fact, simply spending time noticing and thinking about playfulness can make us more playful. The old saying 'where focus

---

30 https://link.springer.com/referenceworkentry/10.1007/978-3-319-24612-3_1885

31 https://iaap-journals.onlinelibrary.wiley.com/doi/full/10.1111/aphw.12220

goes, energy flows' is true. When we focus on playfulness, we will encourage more of it in our lives.

Today we're going to see how we can cultivate a sense of playfulness in our sexual selves.

CURIOSITY

To start

Think of three playful things that have happened recently, either that you were involved in or you witnessed. Write about them in your journal.

Main exercise

Think about the ways you are playful in your non-sexual life, and write about these in your journal. Now, think about some other ways you could be more playful.

Think about the ways you are playful in your sexual life – in both self-pleasure and partnered sex. Now think about some other ways you could be more playful.

SENSATION

With playfulness in mind, try a self-pleasure session inspired by one of the following. As always, begin with Before Care and end with After Care.

MAKE LOVE TO THE EARTH

Become an eco-sexual like my heroine Annie Sprinkle and her wife Beth Stephens.

Marry the Earth and make love to it.

Let this idea inspire you in whatever way you wish. Put a plant by your bed and meditate on it as you masturbate. Commune with the stars, dive into a lake. Show your love for the Earth with dance, song, stroking, or humping in nature.

GET KINKY

The world of kink awaits you, and it really is a world of play. Everyone's kinky looks different – how will you find yours? You might want to purchase some kink kit – perhaps nipple clamps, a scratch claw or a butt plug. Or you might like to explore the contents of your home with a kinky eye . . .

Try finishing the question 'How would it feel if I . . . ?' thinking about household objects: How would it feel if I pressed the shower jet to my genitals? How would it feel if I got my hairbrush and rubbed it all over me? How would it feel if I smacked my mons with that wooden spoon?

TOYS

There is a *huge* sex toy market out there. If you have the money, you might like to explore it: 'I wonder what it would feel like to try that vibrator/dildo/wand/air tickler /crystal egg . . .' etc.

THE ELEMENTS

The elements of water, fire, earth and air can be used playfully. You could bring these elements into the quality of touch you give – e.g. strokes that are warming, like fire – or use the actual elements. Water can be used in so many ways, like erotic washing or bathing or using shower heads, as I mentioned earlier. Air can be interpreted in different ways too: how does it feel when your hairdryer blows on your clitoris? Air carries soundwaves – how about experimenting with different genres of music during self-pleasure and/or lovemaking?

ROLE PLAY

This can be a fun one: who do you want to be? A super-hero, a sports star, a Viking? Do you have anything in your wardrobe you could use as a costume? Props can be fun, too.

ROPE-PLAY

You can play with rope bondage with another person or on yourself. Shibari is the art of tying up a person in a way that looks attractive, making patterns with the ropes you use, and it's known to be an erotic, meditative way to connect with yourself or a partner. Try making yourself a self-tie corset – there are lots of tutorials online.

IMPACT PLAY

Paddles, canes, whips, spanking with the hand. Flog-gers can be fun solo as well as with a partner. They can tickle, stroke and thwack. And how about a feather tickler or fur mitt for after?

DIRTY DANCING

How does it feel to twerk? To pole dance? To do a strip-tease?

YOUR SURRENDER

Here we look at ways we can relax our bodies and minds so that sex can enter the realm of the extraordinary.

DAY 26

I am surrender

If I go into my softness, the soft power of the feminine,
my entire body is orgasmic – we have so many erogenous
zones. But it is less a 'getting to' and more a 'relaxing
into', an arriving into something that already is, which
you make more alive within you.

Odile, Netherlands

One thing that became apparent when I was interviewing women for *Women on Top of the World* was that the women who were *loving* the sex they were having weren't actually thinking at all. Rather than thinking, they were actually feeling.

Less satisfying sex tended to be characterised by worries about appearance and performance, or resentment directed at a partner. But sex that entered the realm of the extraordinary was devoid of thought, and the language women used to describe it was all about sensation: they spoke about floating, expanding, being in the stars, feeling warmth, vibration, softness and calm.

How easy it is for us to surrender to sensation, to let go of everything and just be in the moment, opening ourselves to a full-bodied orgasmic state, is going to be different for all of us. It will also vary for each of us from day to day and over the course of our lives.

'Do I smell?', 'Am I taking too long to come?', 'Did I lock the back door?' – our busy minds can certainly disrupt our capacity to surrender to sensation. But so too can tension in the body.

I was unable to enjoy sex for many, many months after I gave birth. I'd been under the impression that I would be raring to go sexually after six weeks, because the internet informed me I 'should' be. However, while I enjoyed what you might call foreplay, my vagina said a loud 'no' to penetration. I felt as though I wanted my partner's penis inside me, but when my partner and I tried, it was painful and uncomfortable, and all arousal dissipated.

At the time I thought I had a problem, but actually my body was being sensible and simply trying to keep me safe. The birth had been pretty traumatic: a blue-light ambulance ride, then forceps, then I was cut and stitched. Afterwards, when a penis tried to enter, my vagina was quite rightly saying, 'Nothing is coming in here, mate, shit got real last time.' Sex practitioners call this 'genital armouring': a process whereby unconscious guarding patterns can lead to pain, discomfort and numbness during sex.

I learned that I had to encourage a de-armouring process. To do this I simply spent time tenderly touching the area, particularly where my stitches were, and breathing. I cried a fair bit doing this, but fairly soon the whole area was able to feel pleasure again. Now, I try to offer myself a de-armouring practice at least once a year. A lot goes on there that may not feel mindful or loving – mooncup and tampon insertions, a coil being fitted, smear tests and other medical procedures, and of course sex that feels too much.

CURIOSITY

Answer the following question in your journal.

What thoughts do you tend to have during sex?
Do these thoughts add to, or detract from, your sexual
  enjoyment?

SENSATION

Do your Before Care routine. Prepare your space, body, mind and spirit.

1. Incredibly Slow and Mindful Masturbation

How slow can you go? Challenge yourself to have the slowest ever self-pleasure or partnered sex session. Make it the slowest, most mindful sex you have ever had. Focus on the senses: on what you can see, touch, hear, taste, smell. If you notice yourself speeding up, stop and take some long, sensual exhales, then bring your attention back to whatever is very slowly happening.

After Care

Spend some time in stillness.

Be curious. Notice how you feel in your body.

Notice if any thoughts pop into your mind. Don't try to change anything. There is no right or wrong. Simply notice them.

Now journal on (or think about) the following questions:

How was that experience for me?
How am I feeling in this moment?
What do I need right now?

If you are able to, in a slow and mindful way, offer yourself some of what you need.

#2 De-armouring

Choose the right time for this, and make sure you have lots of time to journal and cuddle yourself afterwards, to honour yourself and this practice.

This is similar to Yoni Massage – in fact, you may have experienced some de-armouring effects during that too.

Do your Before Care routine. Now, take the time to simply apply a gentle touch to the external and internal areas of your genitals. Place an oiled finger(s) gently on an area of your genitals and take about ten slow breaths before moving your finger(s) to another point. Send love and tenderness to that area. Use your intuition to guide you where to touch and how much pressure to use. Various emotions may – or may not – arise. Keep breathing. Take the practice very gently.

After Care

Spend some time in stillness.

Be curious. Notice how you feel in your body.

Notice if any thoughts pop into your mind. Don't try to change anything. There is no right or wrong. Simply notice them.

Now journal on (or think about) the following questions:

How was that experience for me?
How am I feeling in this moment?
What do I need right now?

If you are able to, in a slow and mindful way, offer yourself some of what you need.

YOUR
SACREDNESS

It's time for us to be open to the idea that sex can be a mystical experience, which can stir in us feelings of awe and wonder and even provoke a sense of one-ness with the Divine.

DAY 27

I am mysticism

I say, 'Oh, God' a lot. It is really interesting that we say, 'Oh, God' during sex. It's like the biggest, widest set of beingness that we are trying to speak to because we are in such a state of expanded aliveness.

Rehana, UK

The Oxford Languages dictionary defines the word 'mystical' as 'having a spiritual symbolic or allegorical significance that transcends human understanding; inspiring a sense of spiritual mystery, awe, and fascination; concerned with the soul or the spirit, rather than with material things'. Perhaps the saddest part about patriarchal religions policing female sexuality is the loss of education around, and belief in, the ways that sex can feel mystical, sacred and transcendent.

My Catholic upbringing and convent education led me to believe that sex was unholy. The holy women who taught me had made vows of chastity, and the only woman I was told to worship was said to be a virgin, even though she'd had a child. I got the clear impression that sex took you *away* from God, not towards Him.

But when I started to really explore my sexuality, the opposite felt true. My sexual awakening was also a spiritual awakening. The more I explored my own pleasure, the more I found myself having experiences that seemed inexplicable, like the three-day orgasm with the message, or the yoni massage my partner gave me, which had me in floods of tears remembering the abortion I'd had fifteen years before, and talking to the spirit of the daughter I didn't keep.

Rather than taking me away from God, it felt like sex was taking me closer to Him – or Her or Them. And rather than them scolding me, they were embracing me, drying my tears and saying, 'What took you so long?'

My masturbation used to be furtive; I'd be fully dressed, sitting in front of my laptop waiting for a site to load, while adverts popped up on my screen. Now I see self-pleasure more as a form of prayer – to myself, to life and to love. I believe that everything – my body, my sex, my breath, my pleasure, my experience – is holy.

CURIOSITY

Write about the following in your journal.

Describe your spiritual self in a few words or sentences.

What experiences have you had that you could describe as mystical?

Have you had any sexual experiences that you felt were mystical?

SENSATION

The wonderful exercise that follows was offered by my friend, fellow author, priestess and somatic educator, Kay Louise Aldred. It is an invitation to make love with the Divine. Now this may sound completely out there to some readers, and, as ever, it is an invitation which you can always decline. But before you do that perhaps first see if there is a way to amend the exercise so you are comfortable in giving it a try.

Now, the Divine will mean different things to each of

us, some might have a firm sense of a God, Goddess, Angel or Spirit. But you could equally think of the Divine simply as Light or Love.

Make Love with the Divine

The intention here is to unite sexually with the Divine.

As ever, follow your Before Care practice.

Create a safe space for yourself. Light a candle. Speaking aloud, welcome your benevolent being, whom you trust fully and know is unconditionally loving. If this feels too much, then call in Light or Love.

Imagine yourself lying in a bubble of golden light. This is the light of pure love. This bubble holds you in a safe space throughout the practice – and only love and the Divine can enter.

Set the intention to make love with the Divine, so you can experience all the love that is manifested. Begin to self-pleasure. Feel the points of contact of your body against the bed, floor or ground. Invite the Divine into your love bubble.

The Divine is now your lover. Ask the Divine to touch you.

The Divine is pure love, so their touch is the most exquisite touch you will ever have experienced. The Divine is a skilled lover of humanity, and knows exactly how to touch your body. How does your body respond to divine touch? Where are you touched? Why? What are you learning?

Ask the Divine to offer you the deep penetrative experience of Light so that you can understand your human and divine self – and so you can feel the truth that you are a sacred human and that your flesh and the Divine are one.

Keep breathing. Notice how the Divine honours your capacity, never pushing you too far, and is respectful and loving. Be aware of any transcendent or cosmic experiences you are having.

Keep holding the intention: *I am making love with the Divine.* Notice – at the point of orgasm and just afterwards – how your body reacts to this lovemaking. Stay in the love bubble throughout the practice, and your period of integration and reflection, until you feel complete.

Think about the experience. How would you describe it? Thank the Divine and close the bubble.

After Care

Spend some time in stillness.

Be curious. Notice how you feel in your body. Notice if any thoughts pop into your mind. Don't try to change anything. There is no right or wrong. Simply notice them.

Now journal on (or think about) the following questions:

How was that experience for me?
How am I feeling in this moment?
What do I need right now?

If you are able to, in a slow and mindful way, offer yourself some of what you need.

CREATIVITY

Explore, through whatever art form you wish, the idea of sex being mystical, sacred and transcendent. You could choose a visual art form (like painting, drawing or collage), words (poetry, a story or song), dance, or any other format that speaks to you.

YOUR VISION

In this part we see ourselves as playing a role in the great journey of female sexual emancipation. We create a vision of a better tomorrow and start taking baby steps towards it.

I am hope

You must ask for what you really want. Don't go back to sleep!

Rumi

So here we are, at the end of our 28 days together. I wish we could have a cuppa, you and me. I'd move all the books off my chair for you, make you all cosy with a blanket, and invite you to tell me how this has been for you. If you were open to it, I'd love to give you a hug.

Thank you for picking up this book and for trusting me with this precious part of you. I hope this book has been of value to you, and that you've had sensual, playful experiences and pleasure from it. Here's to pleasure!

Female sexuality has had such a tragic time. So many awful things have happened to women, and continue to happen. Women are still shamed, blamed, hurt and killed for being sexual. They have their genitals cut because some people are afraid of the idea of women being free, powerful, joyful and sexual. Across the world, unfair laws and ridiculous myths about female sexuality still abound. But from these ashes we are the phoenix rising – and that is something to be proud of.

We're the trailblazers for a new way. We're creating a new era for sexuality, one where healing, pleasure, sensuality, spirituality, communication, playfulness and creativity are paramount.

It may be a sombre way to end a sex book, but now I'd like us to take a moment to think about all those women who didn't survive, those who lost their lives to violence, those burned or stoned or killed by family members. We're all connected. Their stories have become our stories, and feed our determination to make a better tomorrow.

As we do this work of female sexual reclamation, I feel that we are being supported by the generations of women who couldn't. They see all we are doing, the patterns we are breaking, the healing we are experiencing, the rights we are claiming, and they cheer us on from the spirit world.

Let's whisper our dreams and our hearts' longings to them, and ask them to help us to take the necessary steps to make these dreams reality.

Why?

Because the world needs our beautiful dreams.

DAY 28

CURIOSITY

Spend some time thinking about the 28-day journey you have been on. In your journal, write about what you have discovered, your breakthroughs, and what felt good. Write your words of hope, or a prayer, for the future of female sexuality.

Take time to slow down and breathe. Perhaps you could do the Light Activation Meditation or the Bliss Touch practice. You might like to start with the words 'I wish for . . .' or 'I pray that . . .' Include your hopes and dreams for the generations yet to come, and for all of us alive now – and of course for yourself.

SENSATION

There are three exercises for this last day.

#1 State your Vision

Take your prayer or speech of hope to somewhere beautiful, meaningful or special. Say aloud the words you have written. Mark the occasion in whatever way you wish.

#2 Do One Thing Today to Support the Cause of Sexual Emancipation

For example, you could:
- Share some positive words or images, or start a conversation on social media.
- Donate to a charity, or support a movement that helps girls and young women. This could be stopping female genital mutilation or sexual violence, or promoting sex education or the rights of LGBTQIA+ communities.
- Help educate the young people in your life. Be a safe

place where they can discuss sex and sexuality.

- Share inspiring and thought-provoking material on the subject – YouTube clips, social media posts, books, TV shows, articles, etc.
- Send words of love and encouragement to the people you feel are doing great work in this area. Your support can be profoundly encouraging. Let's be allies to each other, calling each other in, not out.

#3 Give Yourself a Golden Hour of Self-love

Pick and mix from the practices in this book, and others you may know, to give yourself a nourishing, sensual hour (longer, if you can!). Some practices you might like to choose from are:

- Slow Down and Breathe
- Bliss Touch
- Light Activation Meditation
- Waking Up the Hands
- Doing One Thing Super-Slow
- Shaking
- Dancing
- Breast Massage
- Intuitive Touch
- 100 Breaths to Ecstasy

YOUR SEXUAL SELF

- Yoni Breathing
- Vulva Gazing
- Yoni Massage
- Sex Magic Ritual
- Journaling
- Self-pleasure with Fantasy
- Self-pleasure with Erotic Content
- Think Yourself Off
- Incredibly Slow and Mindful Masturbation
- Orgasmic Meditation
- De-armouring
- Make Love with the Divine

Repeat as often as you can. Rule out the time in your diary.

Claim your pleasure.

THE 28 MANTRAS

1. I AM LOVE

2. I AM PEACE

3. I AM SAFETY

4. I AM PLEASURE

5. I AM FLESH

6. I AM SOVEREIGNTY

7. I AM GRATITUDE

8. I AM WISDOM

9. I AM REVERENCE

10. I AM SEX

11. I AM POWER

12. I AM MAGIC

13. I AM DEVOTION

14. I AM SENSATION

15. I AM CONNECTION

16. I AM AROUSAL

17. I AM ACTIVATION

18. I AM EXCITEMENT

19. I AM DISCERNMENT

20. I AM FANTASY

21. I AM EROTICISM

22. I AM DESIRE

23. I AM YES and I AM NO

24. I AM DOMINANCE
and I AM SUBMISSION

25. I AM PLAYFULNESS

26. I AM SENSATION

27. I AM MYSTICISM

28. I AM HOPE

A FINAL THOUGHT

I have a vision. It is a place, a temple, that I have been to many times in my spiritual practice. It is somewhere women go to sit in quiet contemplation as the sun rises and sets. They appear from different places and from their busy lives, wrapping shawls around their shoulders, finding their spots on the ground or temple steps to silently greet and release the day. They take the time each day to see the horizon, the bigger picture, the wonder of it all.

Inside the temple it can be busy or hushed, depending on what's occurring. You'll likely hear women singing and laughing, children playing, soft voices speaking, but there could well be weeping or wailing too.

You might witness a party for a girl's first menstruation. Fresh flowers decorate her hair and scented oils are applied to her feet and hands. Guests eat a feast with fruit and cake. Or perhaps you'll observe a lesson being taught to the younger women in the mysteries of the female body – the ecstasy of breath, touch and time.

This is a place where the body, the sensual and the sexual, is known to be sacred, where its magic and its secrets are taught, and where its cycles of life and death are celebrated and mourned. Women come here to learn and pray, to be in community or to seek counsel. When necessary, this is where they take their sorrow and where they come to heal.

You might see a mother run to the temple with her daughter, tears on both their faces. The girl has been raped. They come to this place of sanctuary to scream and cry, to bathe and sleep, talk and weep. Here they know they will be understood and tended to with love. You may notice a group of elders huddled together, talking earnestly, then leaving the temple to confront the assailant and speak to the community.

This is the Temple of the Divine Feminine. Here, God is a woman. She has as many faces as the women who visit and serve Her, as many faces as the moon and the sun.

I feel that my mission is to bring my vision of this temple to Earth somehow. This book, and the journey in it, is a very small attempt to do just that.

Thank you for being part of this journey.

With so much love

Lucy x

FURTHER READING

MY BOOKS

Don't Hold My Head Down, Unbound, 2019.

Women on Top of the World: What women think about when they are having sex, Quercus, 2021.

Here is a list of all the books I have mentioned in this book and which inspired me, in case you'd like to read them for yourself:

Meggan Watterson, *Mary Magdalene Revealed: The first apostle, her feminist gospel and the Christianity we haven't tried yet*, Hay House, 2019.

Bessel van der Kolk, *The Body Keeps the Score*, Penguin, 2015.

Betty Martin, *The Art of Receiving and Giving: The wheel of consent*, Luminaire Press, 2021.

Sonya Renee Taylor, *The Body Is Not an Apology: The power of radical self-love*, Berrett-Koehler Publishers, second edition, 2021.

Peter Lovatt, *The Dance Cure: The surprising secret to being smarter, stronger, happier*, Short Books Ltd, 2020.

Regena Thomashauer, *Pussy: A reclamation*, Hay House, 2016.

David Bedrick, *You Can't Judge a Body by its Cover: 17 women's stories of hunger, body shame, and redemption*, Belly Song Press, 2020.

Casper Ter Kuile, *The Power of Ritual: Turning everyday activities into soulful practices*, William Collins, 2020.

Nimko Ali, *What We're Told Not to Talk About (But We're Going to Anyway): Women's voices from East London to Ethiopia*, Penguin, 2020.

Barbara Carrellas, *Urban Tantra: Sacred sex for the twenty-first century*, Ten Speed Press, 2017.

Emily Nagoski, *Come As You Are: The surprising new science that will transform your sex life*, Scribe, 2015.

Jack Morin, *The Erotic Mind: Unlocking the inner sources of passion and fulfilment*, Harper Perennial, 2012.

Jan Day, *Living Tantra: A journey into sex, spirit and relationship*, Watkins Publishing, 2021.

Kay Louise Aldred, *Making Love with the Divine: Sacred, ecstatic and erotic experiences*, Girl God Books, 2023.

HELPFUL ORGANISATIONS AND RESOURCES

During this process as you are exploring and getting to know yourself, it may be that you uncover some physical, emotional or sexual issue or trauma which you decide you need more support with. I've included some organisations and resources here that may be of use if this is the case, as well as some more general mental health sign-posting. I really hope you find the support and help you need on your healing journey.

TALK-BASED THERAPY

The British Association for Counselling and Psychotherapy has a directory of therapists, listing counsellors and psychotherapists, if you would like to have private one-to-one talk-based therapy to explore any issues that are affecting you.
https://www.bacp.co.uk

MORE BODY-BASED THERAPIES

Sexological Bodywork® is 'a body-based educational modality that supports individuals, couples and groups to learn to direct their erotic development and to deepen their erotic wellbeing and embodiment'.
https://sexologicalbodyworkers.org/practitioners#!directory/ord=rnd

Somatic Experiencing® is 'a pioneering body-based approach to overcoming trauma, shock and other stress disorders'.
https://www.seauk.org.uk

CHARITIES AND ORGANISATIONS THAT PROVIDE SUPPORT AND ADVICE

BIRTH TRAUMA ASSOCIATION

This organisation provides support for those who have experienced birth trauma.
https://www.birthtraumaassociation.org.uk

BROOK

Brook offers tons of help and advice on sexual health and well-being.
https://www.brook.org.uk

NAPAC

The National Association for People Abused in Childhood has a free, confidential support line and email service and lots of resources online.
https://napac.org.uk

RAPE CRISIS

Rape Crisis offers help and support to victims of rape and sexual violence, no matter when it happened. It has a 24/7 rape and sexual support helpline and a free online chat service, as well as free support, including counselling, group work and other therapies from their local centres. **https://rapecrisis.org.uk/get-help/**

RELATE

Relate's website contains lots of relationship and sex advice. Relate also offers paid-for counselling, online or face to face. **https://www.relate.org.uk/get-help**

THE SURVIVORS TRUST

The Survivors Trust offers advice for survivors of sexual abuse. This includes a free helpline, a live chat service, and information about local services.
https://www.thesurvivorstrust.org

The Survivors Trust Resources website is full of practical resources and self-help tips.
https://www.tstresources.org

THE VAGINISMUS NETWORK

A community for people with vaginismus.
https://www.thevaginismusnetwork.com

VULVAL PAIN SOCIETY

This organisation provides resources, practical advice and information for people living with vulval pain.
https://vulvalpainsociety.org

MENTAL HEALTH SUPPORT

You can refer yourself to talking therapies such as cognitive behaviour therapy and eye movement desensitisation and reprocessing (EMDR) online by looking for your local services on the NHS website.
https://www.nhs.uk/service-search/mental-health/find-an-nhs-talking-therapies-service

The charity MIND offers information and support to people experiencing problems with their mental health.
https://www.mind.org.uk/

MIND also has an extensive list of help available for those who have experienced abuse.
https://www.mind.org.uk/information-support/guides-to-support-and-services/abuse/

SOME PRACTICAL BOOKS FOR MENTAL HEALTH SUPPORT

The Happiness Trap by Russ Harris (second edition, Robinson, 2022) is all about acceptance and commitment therapy. The gist is that life is full of struggles we have no control of, but we can live with these, engage in the here and now, unhook ourselves from painful thoughts and behave in accordance with our values.

The Compassionate Mind Workbook (Chris Irons and Elaine Beaumont, Robinson, 2017) is a book for people with high levels of shame and guilt. It helps readers to develop self-compassion, give compassion and receive compassion, and is based on compassion-focused therapy.

If you are struggling with your mental health, you could ring your GP or contact the Samaritans on 116 123. If you are having a mental health crisis and feel that you can't keep yourself safe, please go to A&E or call an ambulance.